# JAICO B
## BABY NAMES

# JAICO BOOK OF BABY NAMES
## (NAAMAANKIT)

**M.V. Kamath**

# JAICO PUBLISHING HOUSE
MUMBAI • DELHI • BANGALORE • HYDERABAD
KOLKATA • CHENNAI • AHMEDABAD

© M.V. Kamath

All rights reserved. Neither this book nor any part
may be reproduced or transmitted in any form or
by any means, electronic or mechanical, including
photocopying, microfilming, and recording, or by
any information storage or retrieval system,
without prior permission in writing from the
publisher.

JAICO BOOK OF BABY NAMES
(Naamaankit)
ISBN 81-7224-063-5

First Jaico Impression : 1988
Tenth Jaico Impression : 2000
Eleventh Jaico Impression : 2003

*Published by:*
Jaico Publishing House
121, M.G. Road,
Mumbai-400 023

*Printed by :*
Efficient Offset Printers
215, Shahzada Bagh, Industrial ComPlex
Phase-II, Delhi-110035

# Preface

I have always been intrigued by and interested in names. A name gives us an identity. Unlike Ulysses who said he was No-man, the rest of us have names to which we respond. Without names, we are truly nobodies. Which is why I find Shakespeare somewhat unacceptable when he says: What's in a name? that which we call a rose by any other name would smell as sweet. No doubt it would. The premise may be true. But only the word 'rose' is evocative of a fragrance that belongs only to it. A rose, God help us, is a rose, is a rose.

There is a certain magic which we associate with names. Consider the word Raam. It is associated with an **avatar** of Vishnu. We consider Mahatma Gandhi a truly liberated soul indeed because, in the very last breath of his life, even as he fell a victim to a foul bullet, he uttered the words "He Raam!". Try substituting some other word for 'Raam' Any word. The impact is just not the same. 'He Raam' says it all.

So words have meaning and names are words with special meaning attached to them. Even dogs and other animals respond to names. Perhaps they recognise only the sound of the word. But no matter. The sound is animated by life. And a name is life.

This book is an exercise in getting down to names. I find to my infinite regret that I have barely scratched the surface insofar as the totality of the task is concerned. I have stuck only to names largely of Sanskrit origin. And even here the list is maddeningly incomplete. Every day I come across a new name that I know is not included in this list and I am affected by a momentary pang of regret. But I know that there will be more editions of this book and I will catch up with the names that have escaped me. Readers are invited to submit their own lists and they will be gratefully accepted. Hopefully they will provide the meaning of the names as well.

In some societies names recur every third generation. Indeed, it is almost mandatory to give the grandson in a family the name of the deceased grandfather, the grand-daughter, the name of the deceased grandmother. In some other societies this is considered inauspicious. The same name is not repeated at all in yet other societies. Again there was a time when the names of Gods and Goddesses were popular. Raam, Krishna, Narayana, Vishnu, Shiva, Rudra, Brahma, or Laxmi, Saraswati, Radha, Parvati, Durga are even today found among all classes and castes throughout India.

Simultaneously 'secular' names too, have been popular down the ages, names like Mohan and Manohar, Ravi, Surya, Chandra. Kamala, Vimala or Moti, Jawahar, Prem, and Vrinda. It is my contention that the most romantic and the most euphonic and melodious names are to be found in our sanskrit classics, names like Shakuntala and Priyamvada, Damayanti and Nala. Names in Bengali are perhaps the most pleasing. It is hard to find a Bengali name that does not ring bells in the heart.

While some names will never get out of style, some others have sadly fallen by the wayside. As long as there is an India there will always be a Rama, Krishna, Hari Govind and Gopala, Shyama, Madhava, Laxmi, Saraswati and Radha. They may be used singly or in combinations such as Ramkrishna, Gopalakrishna, Harindra, Shyamasunder, Laxminarayan and Chandrashekhar. But these fashions occur in cycles. Today the fashion is not only for secular names, but for short names as well. Anil, Sunil, Rita, Rekha, Lekha, Taru and Sheela are in. Parameshwari, Vasantasena or Chandravadan seem to be out. But they will come back again.

I had a friend who strictly disapproved of certain kinds of names, not because they were ugly but because they placed an unnecessary burden on children. Not every Vidyasagar will turn out to be a scholar, nor every Sunderamurthi a handsome figure. Such names may indicate parental hopes and desires but not filial reality.

In India it is somewhat easy to identify the region one comes from, from the name one bears. A Venkateswaran has to come from Tamil Nadu and an Anantapadmanabhan can only come from the deep south, whether it is Tamil Nadu, Karnataka or Kerala. A Satyajit or an Abanindranath has to come from Bengal, just as a Cariappa, Thimayya or Ramanna has to come from Coorg. But increasingly today the tendency is to erase all signs of regionalism. Thus Ram Kumar, Krishna Kumar or Dilip Kumar blur regional or caste origins. They have become convenient masks for many who want to be known for what they are and not for where they come from. The suffix 'Kumar', like 'Nath', 'Chandra', 'Prasad', etc., override caste and regional distinction.

Parents, again, tend to name their children after celebrities. There must have been many Mohans named around the early twenties after Mahatma Gandhi who shot to fame about that time. How many would be the Indians named after Indira Gandhi and later her sons Rajiv and Sanjay? A survey might lead to some interesting conclusions.

Naming a child is an art by itself. The more culturally sophisticated the parents, the more fanciful would be the names they pick up for their children. Most names are familiar ones: Shankar, Vittal, Ramesh, Suresh, Satish, Ganesh like Raama, Laxmana, Sita and Savitri, pleasing in themselves, are commonplace. Some parents are superstitious about naming their daughters after Ahalya or Draupadi, Sita or Tara, considering how much suffering they have undergone. They do not want their pain visited on their children.

Some names do not have any appeal at all. Mandodari, wife of the demon-king Ravana is mentioned among the **pancha-kanyas** the invocation of whose name is enough to wipe out even **maha patakas** — cardinal sins. And yet whoever has heard of a child being christened as Mandodari? And yet she was a dutiful, husband-worshipping princess, a proper **Bharatiya naari.** Even Urmila, Laxmana's wife is not so common a name as one would suppose. Unlike Sita who accompanied her Lord and master in exile, Urmila stayed behind and did not accompany Laxmana. The Raamayana might have been more complicated had she joined the trio and was in turn kidnapped.

Some names have perennial appeal, names like Ganesh and Gauri. An Arjun is popular but not Bhima. One encounters few Yudhistiras and Dharmarajs but perhaps more Nakulas and Sahadevas, especially in North India.

The nearest English equivalent for **samskaras** is Sacraments. They are rituals and sacrifices, by virtue of performing which the life of a Hindu receives a higher sanctity. **Samskaras** cover his entire life from the moment he is conceived till his death, inclusive of his funeral ceremonies and further on for the smooth passage of his soul to another world.

The sage Angiras said of **samskaras**: "Just as a picture is painted with various colours, so the character of the individual is formed by the proper performance of the **samskaras.**"

**Samskaras** are forty in number, but for the purpose of this book we may refer only to **garbadhana, pumsavana, seemantha, jatakarma** and **naamakarana** — that is from conception to the naming ceremony.

The Atharva Veda contains many prayers for successful conception and childbirth, and for the protection of both mother and child against every kind of danger. Various divinities closely connected with fertility are invoked such as Saraswati and Sinivali (goddess of the new moon and of female fertility) as also the Asvins, Savitr, Dhatr, Tvastr and Prajapati. But it is Angi, the life germ of all creatures, and the power that fecundates the waters, who bestows children.

The **mantras** uttered during the **garbhadaana** ceremony during the **ritu** period of the woman, are essentially prayers offered to God to help the bride conceive a good son. Freely translated they say: "May we produce strong and long-lived sons as fire is produced by friction; may he be well-behaved. I am part of God and I shall produce good sons to liberate my ancestors. May we beget shining, wealthy children. May he donate liberally to the needy and attain **moksha**. May God make you fit for conception. Let the evil spirit flee from you. Let your child be free from defects like lameness, deafness, etc., Be you like the divine **Kaamadhenu**..."

When the husband comes to his wife he says:

> Just as the mighty earth bore the seed of all life
> So may you carry the child and bring forth a son!
> Just as the mighty earth bore the trees of the forests
> So may you carry the child and bring forth a son!

Later he says:

> As the earth bears fire in her womb
> and the heaven is pregnant with lightening
> and the quarters have wind as their seed
> so I place in you, my wife, this child...

There are more prayers on the same lines.

**Pumsavana** ceremony is performed in the second, third or the fourth month of pregnancy. The meaning and object of this ceremony is to "quicken a male child" in the woman. The ceremony is performed on a day of male **nakshatra** (star). In the ritual, a few drops of the juice of the banyan stem are poured into the right nostril of the pregnant lady with a prayer for the birth of a son or a worthy child. A sanctified thread is tied to the left wrist of the lady by way of protection. The **mantras** say: "May God Isana fulfil our wishes; Dhatr bless the world with children and wealth. May He bless this household too with children. May the immortals live in this house. May Agni bless me with sons. May Indra bless me with children. May I have handsome children."

The third in the series of ceremonies of pre-natal **samskaras** is known as **seemantonnayana** and is performed during the period between the fifth and eighth months of pregnancy.

The ceremony derives that name from the parting of the hairs of the pregnant lady at the centre of the head—which is, incidentally, also the etymological meaning of the term. It is said that the parting of the hair symbolises the removal of undesirable shocks to the would-be mother and for keeping her psychologically cheerful and free of care.

The goddess Raka is invoked with a prayer: "I beseech the goddess Raka. May she make this ceremony blameless. May my son be sharp of intellect". Music on the **veena** is expected to be played.

The mother fasts and keeps silent after the ceremony till the rise of the star and at the close of the ceremony, she touches the malf calf, symbolising a son.

The fourth in the series of ceremonies is **jatakarma**. According to the **grihya sutras**, the **jatakarma** proper must be performed before the umbilical cord is severed. The father looks at the face of the new-born babe and at once redeems his debt to his ancestors. It is said that he must immediately bathe in cold water with his clothes on. Actually, he must jump into a river or lake so as to cause the splashing waters rise as high as a palm tree. He is then enjoined to give charity, as the merit earned by him at that time is immense.

Raimundo Panikkar, in his book **The Vedic Experience** quotes from the **Asvalayana Grihya sutra** the ritual to be followed:

At the birth of a son, the child's father, before anyone else touches him, should feed the baby (with a golden spoon) a little butter and honey in which a trace of gold (dust) has been mixed, and say:

> I feed you with the wisdom of honey
> I feed you with ghee, the gift of God, the beautiful,
> May you have long life, protected by the gods,
> May you live in this world a hundred circling years!

Then. putting his lips close to the child's ears, he murmurs:

> May God grant you intelligence
> may His Power grant you intelligence,
> may his two divine Messengers, lotus-wreathed
> grant to you intelligence.

Near the child's naval or right ear he says softly:

> The Lord is full of life:
> through firewood he is full of life
> By this vital power I make you full of life
> The divine Drink is full of life;
> through herbs he is full of life......

He then says a prayer to earth, on the spot in which the child is born:

> I know your heart, O Earth, that rests in heaven,
> in the moon, I know your heart, may it know me!
> May we see a hundred circling years
> may we live a hundred circling years
> may we hear (the sounds of) a hundred years!

He then prays for the strength of the child and touching the child's shoulders, says:

> Be a stone, be an axe, be unsurpassed gold
> You, in truth, are the Veda, called my son.
> Live, therefore, a hundred years
> Powerful God, give us the best of treasures,

Grant us your gifts, O bountiful, O swift One!
Later he calls for an infusion of learning in the child

**Bhuh!**
I instil the Rg Veda into you.
**Bhuvah!**
I instil the Yajur Veda into you...
**Svah!**
I instil the Sama Veda into you.
**Svaha! Bhur, Bhuvah, Svah!**
I instil the Speculations into you,
the history and the Legends into you — Om!
all the Vedas I instil into you...

Finally, he says a prayer for the mother.

You are Ida, the daughter of Mitra and Varuna
You, a courageous woman, have borne a vigorous son.
May you be blessed with vigorous children
You who have blessed us with a vigorous son!

The fifth of the **samskaras** is **naamakarana,** the naming of the child. According to Asvalayana, the names of boys should have an even number of syllables. A two-syllabled name (Raama, Krishna) will bring material fame and four-syllabled, religious fame. The girl's name should have an odd number of syllables and end in 'i' 'ee' or 'as' (Raadhaa, Maitreyee, Rukmini, Kalindi).

The **naamakaran** ceremony is normally performed on the tenth or twelfth day after birth.

After preliminaries, the parent gives the offering to gods, touches the breath of the child symbolishing the awakening of its consciousness and say in its ear: "Your name is...." thrice. Brahmins and elder are then requested to follow, calling the child by its given name and blessing it. In some societies it is customary to place in the palm of the child a gold coin.

I have had much assistance from a number of friends in the compiling of names. The first to set me on my path was Usha Puri who "contributed" a few names as a starter. Dr Kalindi Randeri then suggested Juthika Sanghavi who did most of the spade work and is mainly responsible for the research and card-indexing. I cannot be sufficiently thankful to her for the many hours she put in over several months. She laboriously compiled the names from many sources and has been of inestimable help to me. Much of the credit for this book goes to her. Subsequently I had the text checked and cross-checked by Sumati Modak and my friend and former colleague, R. Gopalakrishna, to both of whom my thanks are due. Special thanks are due to Dr Kalindi Randeri, who, in addition to providing for the infrastructure, also read the proofs and extended many valuable suggestions.

And, of course, if for all the work that has gone in some errors still persist, the fault is entirely mine.


Kalyanpur House,                                                M.V. Kamath
Bombay.

# A

Aabhaa (f) light
Aabhaas (m) awareness
Aabharikaa (f) one who has a halo
Aabhirikaa (f) a cowherd's wife
Aadarsha (m) a looking glass
Aadhikara (m) Shiva
Aadhyaa (f) the first power; one of the ten Durgas
Aadi (m) first
Aadideva (m) the first god
Aadima (m) in the beginning
Aadimurti (m) first creation
Aadinatha (m) the first lord
Aadishwara (m) the first god
Aadisura (m) the first god
Aadita (m) from the first Aaditaa (f)
Aaditi (f) the earth
Aaditteya (m) immortal
Aaditya (m) sun
Aadityanaaraayana (m) sun
Aadityavardhana (m) one who embellishes the sun
Aadityesha (m) the sun god
Aagama(m) coming, birth
Aagneya (m) son of Agni
Aahlaada (m) delight
Aahlaaditaa (f) a woman in a happy mood
Aakaankshaa(f) desire
Aakaashdeepa(m) light of the sky
Aakarsha (m) to attract
Aakasha (m) to shine
Aakil (m) intelligent
Aakraanti (f) might, force

Aakuti (f) desire, intention
Aalaapa (m) first part of a dialogue
Aalaapee (m) one who sings
Aalaapini (f) a songstress
Aalambi (m) hold on to
Aalochana (m) to perceive
Aaloka (m) cry of victory
Aalokaa (f) woman having lustre
Aamodini (f) fragrance
Aamrakali (f) bud of the mango tree
Aamramanjari (f) blossom of the mango tree
Aamrapali (f) leaf of the mango tree
Aamrapallavi (f) as above
Aanana (m) visage; face
Aananandamaya (m) steeped in happiness
Aananda (m) joy
Aanandabrahma (m) eternal joy
Aanandagiri (m) mountain of joy
Aanandamurti (m) picture of happiness
Aanandaparnaa (f) one having wings of joy
Aanandarupa (m) eternal joy
Aanandasaagara (m) sea of joy
Aanandaswarupa (m) eternal joy
Aanandavardhana (m) one who adds to joy
Aanandi (f) always happy

1

**Aanandini** (f) giver of joy

**Aananditaa** (f) one who spreads joy

**Aandola** (m) to swing, moving

**Aanetra** (m) to see until one is satisfied

**Aapta** (m) reliable, trustworthy

**Aapti** (f) fitness, completion

**Aaraa** (f) decorative

**Aaraadhaka** (m) one who worships **Aaraadhikaa** (f)

**Aarohee** (f) a creeper

**Aarunaka** (m) reddish

**Aarunamshu** (f) reddish rays

**Aarunikaa** (f) tawny red

**Aaryadeva** (m) best among the Aryans

**Aaryashura** (m) courageous

**Aasha** (f) hope

**Aashaalataa** (f) creeper of hope

**Aashaankita** (m) full of hope

**Aashika** (m) lover

**Aashikaa** (f) beloved

**Aashisha** (f) blessed woman

**Aashitendu** (m) satisfied by eating

**Aashlesha** (m) to embrace

**Aashtika** (m) son of the sage Jaratharu and his wife Manasa devi

**Aashutosha** (m) one who is easily pleased

**Aasmitaa** (f) egoism egotism

**Aastika** (m) one who has faith in the Vedas

**Aatiteya** (m) son of Aatit

**Aatmaananda** (m) one who has won victory over one's self

**Aatmadeva** (m) soul

**Aatmaja** (m) born to oneself

**Aatmajaa** (f) daughter of the mountain

**Aatman** (m) the self

**Aatmaram** (m) one who strives to get spiritual knowledge

**Aatmayu** (m) one blessed with long life

**Aayati** (m) majestic, dignified

**Aayu** (m) span of life

**Aayushmaan** (m) one blessed with long life

**Abhaya** (m) fearless **Abhayaa** (f)

**Abhayadatta** (m) son of the fearless

**Abhayasimha** (m) fearless lion

**Abhi** as a prefix to verbs and nouns: in the direction of, against, over, near, before

**Abhichandra** (m) an auspicious time

**Abhijaata** (m) noble, wise

**Abhijaya** (m) one who is victorious **Abhijit** (m)

**Abhijitaa** (f) a woman conquered

**Abhijita** (m) name of a sage

**Abhijna** (f) expert

**Abhijnya** (m) **recognition Abhijnaa** (f)

**Abhik** (m) lover

**Abhimaanee** (m) one who is proud

**Abhimaneenee** (f) one who is possessed of self respect

**Abhimanyu** (m) quick to anger

**Abhinandaa** (f) one who delights

**Abhinava** (m) quite new

**Abhiraaja** (m) great king

**Abhiraama** (m) pleasing

**Abhiratha** (m) great charioteer

**Abhirupa** (m) beautiful

**Abhirupaa** (f) beautiful woman

**Abhisaarikaa** (f) woman who keeps her tryst with her lover

**Abhisheka** (m) to sprinkle

**Abhishta** (f) one who is dear

**Abhu** (m) unborn

**Abhivaadana** (m) to salute

**Abhivandaka** (f) one who salutes respectfully

**Abhyuday** (m) one who has risen to prosperity

**Abjini** (f) a collection of lotuses

**Achala** (m) one who is steady

**Achalaa** (f) the earth

**Achalatanayaa** (f) daughter of the mountain

**Achalendra** (m) king of the mountains

**Achintya** (m) one who is beyond comprehension

**Achiraa** (f) one who is brief

**Achyuta** (m) indestructable

**Achyutaananda** (m) the joy of remaining steadfast

**Achyutavikranta** (m) courageous

**Adhara** (m) one who is under

**Adheera** (m) impatient

**Adheesha** (m) emperor

**Adheeta** (m) scholar

**Adheip** (m) king

**Adhideva** (m) highest god

**Adhika** (m) more

**Adhvaryu** (m) one who knows how to perform yajnas

**Aditi** (f) boundless

**Adri** (m) mountain

**Adrijaa** (f) daughter of the mountain

**Adrikaa** (f) small mountain

**Advaitaa** (f) a unique woman

**Advaya** (m) unique

**Agendra** (m) king of the mountains

**Aghanaashaa** (f) destroyer of sin

**Aghanaashinee** (f) the godess who destroys sin

**Aghora** (m) not horrible

**Agnajita** (m) conqueror of fire

**Agnayi** (f) goddess of fire

**Agnibhatta** (m) one who has unsubdued splendour

**Agnika** (m) related to fire

**Agnima** (m) leader

**Agrabodhi** (m) the first guru

**Agrajaa** (f) elder daughter

**Agrajeeta** (m) one who wins first

**Aharnisha** (m) day and night

**Airaawata** (m) proceeding from water

**Aishwaryaa** (f) prosperity

**Aja** (m) unborn

**Ajaa** (f) she-goat

**Ajaamila** (m) unfriendly

**Ajaata** (m) unborn

**Ajaatashatru** (m) without enemies

**Ajalaa** (f) the earth

**Ajaya** (m) invincible

**Ajeya** (m) unconquerable

**Ajhati** (f) woman of good character

**Ajinkya** (m) unconquerable

**Ajitaabh** (m) one who has conquered the skies

**Ajitesha** (m) victorious god

**Ajneya** (m) the unknown

**Akalkaa** (f) moonlight

**Akalmasha** (m) one who leads a spotless life

**Akshata** (m) uninjured

**Alolupa** (m) free from desire

**Akhila** (m) entire, whole
**Akhilaa** (f)

**Akshobhya** (m) serene

**Akhshita** (m) immortal

**Akshayamati** (f) immortal woman

**Akshayataa** (f) imperishable

**Akshayini** (f) immortal

**Akshina** (m) infallible

**Akshayee** (f) undecaying

**Akshayakeerti** (m) eternal fame

**Akshajaa** (f) thunderbolt

**Akshina** (m) one who is not feeble

**Akshataa** (f) a virgin

**Akshee** (f) eye

**Aksha** (m) the soul

**Akopa** (m) one who does not get angry

**Akula** (m) Shiva

**Alaka** (f) lock of curly hair

**Akrur** (m) not cruel

**Alarka** (m) able

**Alpa** (m) one who does not disappear

**Alopaa** (f) free from desire

**Alpaa** (f) minute

**Alpanaa** (f) decoration

**Amalaa** (f) without sin

**Amalendu** (m) full moon

**Alpesha** (m) smaller than an atom

**Alakanandaa** (f) a young girl

**Ameya, Amiya** (m) boundless

**Amita** (m) boundless

**Amarajaa** (f) daughter of the gods

**Amaraanganaa** (f) immortal woman

**Amarachandra** (m) eternal moon

**Amaresha** (m) eternal god

**Amaranaatha** (m) immortal lord

**Ambaa** (f) mother

**Ambara** (m) the sky

**Ambujaa** (f) lotus

**Amara** (m) immortal

**Ameetaa** (f) unlimited

**Ameeta** (m)

**Amola** (m) valuable

**Amteshwara** (f) eternal god

**Amitaabha** (m) one with boundless splendour

**Amrutesha** (m) god of nectar

**Amrita** (m) nectar

**Amritaa** (f) immortal

**Ammavasu** (m) wealthy

**Amogha** (m) unerring

**Amula** (m) priceless

**Amitaatma** (m) divine soul

**Amiti** (f) boundless

**Amritamshu** (m) drop of nectar, moon

**Amish** (m) honest

**Amishaa, Amishi** (f)

**Ameya** (m) magnanimous

**Amoghasiddhi** (m) one who does not fail

**Amrrata** (m) nectar

**Amurta** (m) without form

**Amrushaa** (f) absolute truth

**Ambarisha** (m) lord of the sky

**Advaitaa** (f) matchless

**Amitesha** (m) infinite god

**Anaadi** (m) one who has no beginning

**Anagha** (m) innocent
**Anaghaa** (f)

4

**Anamola** (m) invaluable
**Ananga** (m) one without a body
**Anangalekhaa** (f) love letter
**Anangamaalinee** (f) garland of kama
**Anangapaala** (m) protector of Ananga
**Anangasuhrid** (m) friend of Ananga
**Anantaa** (f) eternal
**Anantabhakti** (m) eternal devotion
**Anantaadevee** (f) eternal goddess
**Anantadeva** (m) eternal god
**Anantajeeta** (m) ever victorious
**Anantakrishna** (m) Krishna, the eternal
**Anantapaala** (m) eternal guardian
**Anantaraama** (m) eternal god
**Anantashaktivarman** (m) one who has eternal strength
**Anantashirsha** (m) one with countless heads
**Anantashree** (m) one who has boundless wealth
**Ananyaa** (f) the only one
**Anasuyaa** (f) one without malice
**Anchit** (m) honoured
**Anga** (m) limb
**Anganaa** (f) beautiful woman with well rounded limbs
**Angada** (m) bracelet
**Angadaa** (m) woman wearing a bracelet
**Angajidd** (m) victorious
**Angalekhaa** (f) lekhaa line
**Angavallee** (f) a creeper
**Anjali** (f) homage

**Anjalika** (m) a small house
**Anjanee** (f) one who adorns herself with ointments and sandalwood paste
**Anjasa** (m) honest **Anjasee** (f)
**Anuli** (f) homage
**Anjushree** (f) married woman who adorns herself
**Aneesha** (m) supreme
**Aneeshaa** (f)
**Aneka** (m) many
**Anenaa** (m) faultless
**Aniketa** (m) homeless
**Anila** (m) god of wind
**Anilabha** (m) gentle wind
**Animaa** (f) the power of becoming minute
**Animisha** (m) one who does not wink
**Anirjita** (m) one who is unconquered
**Aniruddha** (m) cooperative
**Anishaa** (f) one in whose life there is no darkness
**Annandaa** (f) goddess of food
**Annapurnaa** (f) same as above
**Amshu** (m) minute particle
**Amshubhadra** (m) beneficial rays
**Amshudhara** (m) the bearer of rays
**Amshuka** (m) muslin
**Amshula** (m) radiant
**Amshumaalaa** (f) garland of rays
**Amshumalina** (m) one who is adorned with rays; the sun
**Amshumaan** (m) the sun
**Amshumanta** (m) adorned with rays
**Amshumati** (f) a radiant woman
**Antariksha** (m) the sky

5

**Antasheelaa** (f) a virtuous woman

**Anu** either used with nouns to form adverbial compounds or as a prefix to verbs or as a separate preposition (after, with, toward, near, like)

**Anubhuti** (f) experience

**Anujnaa** (f) permission

**Anugra** (m) calm

**Anuja** (m) born after

**Anujaa** (f)

**Anshula** (m) radiant

**Anuraaga** (m) devotion, love

**Archishaa** (f) light, flame

**Aryama** (m) the sun

**Ati** a prefix used with adjectives and verbs — 'very'

**Atulya** (m) unequalled

**Auttamikaa** (f) relating to gods who are in the highest place

**Avaneesha, Avaneeshwara** (m) master of the world

**Anulaa** (f) brought up together

**Anulekhaa** (f) born later

**Anulomaa** (f) one who marries a man of a caste higher than herself

**Anumati** (f) permission

**Anumeha** (m) following the rain

**Anupa** (m) a pond

**Anupaa** (f)

**Anupamaa** (m) incomparable

**Anupameya** (m) incomparable

**Anupriyaa** (f) incomparable

**Anusheelaa** (f) devoted servant

**Anuraadhaa** (f) one who is pleased to worship

**Anuraga** (m) attachment

**Anurati** (f) full of affection

**Anuttama** (m) best of all

**Anuttamaa** (f)

**Anuttaraa** (f) one who is unanswered

**Anuvaa** (f) to blow

**Anuvidyaa** (f) to gain through knowledge

**Anuvind** (m) one who has obtained

**Anvitaa** (f) one who bridges the gap

**Anuyaa** (f) woman who follows

**Anviksha** (f) see, gaze

**Aparajita** (m) not conquerable

**Aparajitaa** (f)

**Aparnaa** (f) leafless

**Aparupaa** (f) very beautiful

**Apoorvee** (f) supreme soul

**Apoorva** (m) quite new

**Apekshaa** (f) expectation

**Araamati** (f) a personified Vedic goddess of piety

**Aranyanee** (f) Vedic goddess vegetation, wood sprite

**Arajaa** (f) clean

**Archanaa** (f) one who adores

**Archee** (f) ray, flame

**Archishaa** (f) a ray of light also **Archish** (m)

**Apava** (m) Narayana

**Archit** (m) one who has been honoured **Architaa** (f)

**Arha** (m) deserving

**Arhana** (m) devotee and attendant of Vishnu

**Arhata** (m) one who is venerable

**Arjikaa** (f) one who seeks mercy

**Arjuna** (m) peacock

**Arnava** (m) sea, ocean

**Akalanka** (m) one without sin

**Analaa** (f) goddess of fire

**Antaraa** (f) in the middle

**Arihanta** (m) one who has killed his enemies

**Arijita** (m) same as above

**Arinjaya** (m) same as above

**Arisudana** (m) same as above

**Arka** (m) the sun

**Arpanaa** (f) offering

**Arpitaa** (f) one who is given away

**Aruna** (m) the dawn

**Arunabha** (m) reddish lustre

**Akhandaananda** (m) eternal joy

**Akhilendra** (m) king of the universe

**Akhilesha** (m) lord of the universe

**Aruni** (f) ruddy complexioned

**Arunimaa** (f) reddishness

**Arundhati** (f) morning star

**Arunamshu** (m) one who has red rays

**Aravinda** (m) lotus

**Aravindaa** (f)

**Asaman** (m) light

**Asanga** (m) one who is a loner

**Aseemaa** (f) limitless

**Ashesha** (m) entire

**Ashma** (m) mountain

**Ashmaka** (m) mountain of stone

**Ashnaa** (f) daughter of king Bali

**Atulya** (m) incomparable

**Ashni** (f) flash of lightning

**Ashoka** (m) one who has no sorrow

**Asiknee** (f) a holy river

**Asita** (m) not white

**Asitabaran** (m) dark complexioned

**Ashwatthaamaa** (m) fiery-tempered

**Ashvina** (m) a cavalier

**Ashwinee** (f) first of the 27 nakshatras

**Asmitaa** (f) ego

**Asti** (f) existence

**Atithi** (m) unexpected guest

**Atula** (m) matchless **Atulaa** (f)

**Avaloka** (m) one who beholds

**Avani**(m) the earth

**Avanindra** (m) king of the earth (ava – to protect)

**Avanisha** (m) lord of the earth

**Avanimohana** (m) one who attracts the whole world

**Avanindranatha** (m) king of the earth

**Avanti** (f) name of a city

**Avarodhan** (m) one who observes restraint

**Avinaasha** (m) one who cannot be destroyed

**Avinaashinee** (f)

**Avalokiteshwara** (m) a Bodhisattva ranked almost as high as a god

**Atyaananda** (m) one who brings great pleasure

# B

**Babhravee** (f) another name of Durga

**Baadala** (m) cloud

**Baadaraayani** (m) name of Shuka, son of Vyasa

**Bahak** (m) an inhabitant of Punjab

**Baageshree** (f) beauty

**Baahubala** (m) powerful

**Baahubalee** (m) simple

**Baahulee** (f) full moon in the month of Kartik

**Baalaa** (f) young girl

**Baaladitya** (m) young sun

**Baalagangaadhara** (m) young Shankar

**Baalachandra** (m) young moon

**Baalagovinda** (m) another name for Krishna

**Baalaajee** (m) another name for Vishnu

**Baalakrishna** (m) young Krishna

**Baalamani** (m) young jewel

**Baalamohan** (m) one who is attractive

**Baalasaraswati** (m) young Shankar

**Baalaarjuna** (m) young Arjun

**Baalaarka** (m) rising sun

**Baalagopaala** (m) a cowherd

**Baalindama** (m) one who destroyed Baali

**Baanee** (f) speech

**Baasavaraja** (m) king of wealth

**Baasu** (m) one who is wealthy

**Babhru** (m) deep-brown

**Badarikaa** (f) name of one of the many sources of the Ganges

**Badarinaryana** (m) Narayana whose abode is Badari

**Badarinatha** (m) lord of Badari

**Badariprasaada** (m) gift of Badari

**Bahinaa** (f) sister

**Bajarangbali** (m) derived from Vajra, Indra's thunderbolt

**Balajaa** (f) earth

**Barishmati** (f) a woman bright as fire

**Balabhadra** (m) one with immense strength

**Balasudana** (m) one who has the power to hurt

**Balavant** (m) one who has immense strength

**Bansari** (f) flute

**Bansi** (m) flute

**Bansidhara** (m) one who holds the flute

**Bansilala** (m) son of Bansi

**Batuka** (m) a brahmin youth

**Beeja** (f) origin, seed

**Beejalee** (f) lightning

**Bakula** (m) a kind of tree

**Bakulaa** (f) tiny white flower

**Bali** (m) son of Virochana

**Balaraama** (m) one of the seven sons of Rohini

**Baladeva** (m) godlike in power

**Beenaa** (f) intelligence

8

**Beemala** (m/f) pure, spotless
**Belaa** (f) wave, limit
**Bhaagyaa** (f) prosperity
**Bhaagyalakshmee** (f) Lakshmi who brings prosperity
**Bhaamaa** (f) a passionate woman
**Bhadra** (f) the Ganges
**Bhadramallikaa** (f) beautiful jasmine
**Bhramara** (m) bee
**Bhaminee** (f) beautiful woman
**Bhaagavanti** (f) fortunate woman
**Balendra** (m) lord of light
**Bhaamaha** (m) the sun
**Bhaanavee** (f) daughter of Bhaanu
**Bhaanu** (m) sun, ray of light
**Bhaanushree** (f) handsome woman
**Bhaanudutta** (m) gift of the sun
**Bhaanumatee** (f) beautiful woman
**Bhaanuprasada** (m) gift of the sun
**Bhaanushankara** (m) name of Shiva
**Bharadwaaja** (m) a lucky bird
**Bhaavan** (m) creator
**Bhaavanaa** (f) faith, desire
**Bhaarata Bhushana** (m) a national treasure
**Bhaargava** (m) the perceptor of demons
**Bhaargavee** (f) daughter of the sun
**Bhaasantee** (f) a brilliant woman
**Bhaaskara** (m) the sun
**Bhaasvaan** (m) bright
**Bhaasvara** (m) bright

**Bhaasvanta** (m) full of light
**Bhaasvatee** (f) one who is luminous
**Bhaaratee** (f) goddess of speech
**Bhaavika** (m) natural
**Bhaavikaa** (f)
**Bhaavinee** (f) a noble lady
**Bhadraka** (m) handsome
**Bhadrikaa** (f)
**Bhadraaksha** (m) a man having beautiful eyes
**Bhadraakshee** (f)
**Bhadraayu** (m) man having a happy life
**Bhadramukha** (m) one with a beautiful face
**Bhadramukhee** (f)
**Bhadrasheela** (m) one with a good character
**Bhadrasheelaa** (f)
**Bhadravatee** (f) gentle woman
**Bhadrikaa** (f) woman with good fortune
**Bhadra** (m) beneficial
**Bhadrabaalaa** (f) beautiful young woman
**Bhadradaa** (f) one who brings good fortune **Bhadraka** (m)
**Bhadrakaalee** (f) name of Durga
**Bhadrakaaya** (m) one with a beautiful body
**Bhadrajeeta** (m) one who is victorious
**Bhadraalee** (f) beautiful female friend
**Bhadraanga** (m) fair-limbed
**Bhadrapaala** (m) a good friend ready to give protection
**Bhadraparnaa** (f) having beautiful leaves

**Bhadrapaalita** (m) one who is guarded by a friend

**Bhadrapriyaa** (f) beloved

**Bhadrashravaa** (m) one who has beautiful ears

**Bhagvati** (f/m) a religious woman, goddess

**Bhagavaticharana** (m) at the feet of the goddess

**Bhagavatiprasada** (m) gift of the goddess

**Bhaagyadatta** (m) given by good fortune

**Bhairavee** (f) a classical melody

**Bhakti** (f) devotion

**Bhaktajaa** (f) one born to a religious woman

**Bhagavaana** (m) the lord

**Bhagavaandaasa** (m) servant of the lord

**Bhavaambee** (f) mother of a good woman

**Bharata** (m) universal monarch

**Bharani** (m) constellation

**Bhasmanga** (m) one who smears his body with ashes

**Bhasmaanka** (m) one who has ashes as his symbol, Shiva

**Bhauma** (m) belonging to the earth **Bhaumaa** (f)

**Bhaumika** (m) one who exists on earth

**Bhava** (m) a name for Shiva

**Bhavabhuti** (m) ashes of Shiva

**Bhavadatta** (m) given by Shiva

**Bhavajna** (m) one who has knowledge of the world

**Bhavanaga** (m) serpent of Shiva

**Bhavesha** (m) lord of the world, name of Shiva

**Bhavya** (m) good-featured

**Bhavyattaa** (f) one with regal splendour

**Bheema** (m) fearful

**Bhogavati** (f) one who gives pleasure

**Bholaanaatha** (m) name of Shiva

**Bhramee** (f) full of lustre

**Bhramaanee** (f) Saraswatee

**Bhoomaananda** (m) joy of the earth

**Bhoomeejaa** (f) daughter of the earth

**Bhoominjaya** (m) one who wins the world

**Bhoopen** (m) king

**Bhoopendra** (m) king of kings

**Bhoopata** (m) lord of the earth

**Bhooshana** (m) an ornament

**Bhuvana** (m) any one of three worlds

**Bhuvanesha** (m) lord of the worlds

**Bilvamangala** (m) lucky

**Bimbiikaa** (f) the disc of the sun or moon

**Bimbisaara** (m) a king of the Gupta dynasty

**Binaa** (f) a musical instrument

**Bindiyaa** (f) a droplet

**Bindu** (f) a drop

**Bindumaalini** (f) one wearing a garland of pearls

**Bindumatee** (f) a small particle

**Bindusaara** (m) an excellent pearl

**Bineetaa** (f) one who is humble

**Binoda** (m) one who is amusing

**Biraaja** (m) to shine

**Bipinchandra** (m) moon of the forest

**Birbala** (m) strength of the victorious

**Birendra** (m) king of the courageous

**Bisini** (f) a cluster of lotuses

**Bisvajeeta** (m) conqueror of the world

**Brahma** (m) supreme being

**Brahmaananda** (m) gift of Brahma

**Buddhadeva** (m) a wise person

**Brijamohana** (m) name of Krishna

**Brijesha** (m) lord of the land of Brij

**Brajena** (m) one who lives in Brij

**Brijaraaja** (m) king of Brij

**Buddha** (m) a wise or learned man

**Buddhamitra** (m) friend of the wise

**Buddhidhana** (m) one who possesses a wealth of wisdom

**Bulabula** (f) name of a bird which sings sweetly

# C

Chag (m/f) love
Chaahabaa (f) affection
Chaitanya (m) life, knowledge
Chaitra (m) sixth month of Vikrama samvant and first of Shaalivaahana year
Chaitree (f)
Chakora (m) alert
Chakradhara (m) one who wields the disc
Chakradhaaree (m) Vishnu
Chakrakee (m) potter
Chakreenee (f)
Chakrapaalita (m) protector of the disc
Chakravarti (m) a sovereign
Chakree (m) a universal monarch, Vishnu, Krishna
Chakshu (m) an eye
Chakshumatee (f) eye-sight
Chakshusha (m) related to eyes
Chaalaka (m) one who drives
Chaman (m) garden
Chamaasa (m) a vessel used at sacrifices for drinking the soma juice
Chamelee (f) a creeper with flowers
Champakamaalaa (f) garland of champak flowers
Chamakali (f) an ornament worn by women
Champaa (f) a yellow flower
Champaakalee (f) bud of champa
Champakavelee (f) a creeper with flowers

Champaavarnee (f) one who has the complexion of a champa flower
Chamundaa (f) an aspect of shakti
Chaamundi (f) Durga, killer of demons
Chaanaaksha (m) clever
Chandaamshu (m) the sun
Chanchala (f) unsteady
Chanchalaa (f) lightning
Chaanda (m) moon
Chandaa (f)
Chandaalikaa (f) low-caste woman
Chandana (f/m) sandalwood
Chandanaa (f)
Chaandnee (f) also chandani moonlight
Chandanikaa (f) a small sandalwood tree
Chandanagandhaa (f) one perfumed with sandalwood paste
Chandilaa (f) Chandikaa, wrathful
Chandodeva (m) the moon
Chandra (m) glittering
Chandrabha (m) lustre of moonlight
Chandrabhaala (m) one who wears the moon on his forehead
Chandrabimba (m) reflection of the moon
Chandrahaasa (m) bow of Shiva
Chandraagad (m) Shiva

**Chandradatta** (m) gift of the moon

**Chandragaura** (m) fair like the moon

**Chandragupta** (m) protected by the moon, founder of the Gupta Dynasty

**Chandrajaa** (f) a moonbeam

**Chandraka** (m) the feather of a peacock

**Chandrakalaa** (f) beauty of the moon

**Chandramani** (f) moonstone

**Chandrakeshwara** (m) Shiva

**Chandraketu** (m) son of Lakshmana

**Chandraki** (m) peacock

**Chandrakirana** (m) moonbeam

**Chandrakirti** (m) one whose fame is like the soft rays of the moon

**Chandralekhaa** (f) digit of the moon

**Chandrajyoti** (f) moonlight

**Chandraalee** (f) friend of the moon

**Chandramadhava** (m) sweet

**Chandramaalaa** (f) a garland

**Chandramaasee** (f) wife of Brihaspati

**Chandraamatee** (f) a serene woman

**Chandramohana** (m) attractive like the moon

**Chandramukha** (m) a moonfaced person
**Chandramukhee** (f) a beautiful woman

**Chandraanana** (m) roundfaced **Chandraanani** (f)

**Chandramallikaa** (f) a kind of jasmine flower

**Chandraamshu** (m) moonbeam

**Chandraprakasha** (m) moonlight

**Chandrarekhaa** (f) streak of the moon

**Chandrashekhara** (m) one who holds the moon in his **shekhara** (hair knot)

**Chandrashilaa** (f) soft, gentle

**Chandravadanee** (f) moonfaced

**Chandraavallaree** (f) moon creeper

**Chandravasaa** (f) one who lives on the moon

**Chandraavatee** (f) illuminated by the moon

**Chandraayana** (m) the path of the moon

**Chandresha** (m) king of the moon

**Chandrila** (m) another name of Shiva

**Chandree** (f) moonlight

**Chandrika** (m) **Chandrikaa** (f)

**Chandrama** (m) the moon

**Chandrimaa** (f)

**Chaandavela** (f) a king of creeper

**Chant** (m) lover

**Chantni** (f) beloved

**Chapala** (m) active

**Chapalaa** (f) goddess Laxmi

**Charanjeet** (m) one who has won over the lord

**Charchrikaa** (f) joy, happiness

**Chaarubaalaa** (f) beautiful young girl

**Chaaruchandra** (m) beautiful moon

**Chaaruchitra** (m) beautiful picture

**Chaarudhaara** (f) a beautiful woman

**Chaarudatta** (m) born of beauty

**Chaaruhaasa** (m) one who has a beautiful smile

**Chaaruhassinee** (f)

**Chaarukeshee** (f) one with beautiful long hair

**Chaarulataa** (f) beautiful creeper

**Chaarumatee** (f) one who is endowed with beauty

**Chaaruvaakee** (f) a woman who speaks sweetly

**Chaarusheela** (f) a beautiful woman of good character

**Chandrakirtee** (m) glory

**Chaarvanga** (m) one with beautiful body

**Chaarvee** (f) beautiful

**Chaturaa** (f) one who is cleaver

**Chaturbhuja** (m) one with four hands

**Chaturmukha** (m) one with four faces

**Chaturvyuha** (m) one who personifies four arrays: Vasudeva, Dankarshana, Pradyumna and Aniruddha (Vyuha   a military array)

**Charvanaa** (f) one who reflects

**Chhaayaa** (f) shadow

**Chhayaanka** (m) moon

**Chelakee** (f) nickname (little girl)

**Cheshtaa** (f) joke

**Chetana** (m) supreme soul

**Chetanaa** (f) wisdom

**Chetanaananda** (m) supreme joy

**Chetas** (m) the mind

**Chetohaaree** (m) attractive

**Chhela** (m) a dandy

**Chikitsaa** (f) one who administers medicines

**Chidaabhaasa** (m) the individual soul

**Chidghana** (m) full of knowledge

**Chidambara** (m) one whose heart is as vast as the sky

**Chidaakaasha** (m) universal soul

**Chidaatmaa** (m) supreme spirit

**Chiddhaatu** (m) original soul

**Chidroopa** (m) knowledge incarnate

**Chikirshaa** (f) desire to do something

**Chingee** (f) also **Chingaaree** spark

**Chinmaatra** (m) absolute knowledge

**Chirantanaa** (m) ancient

**Chirapushpa** (m) the bakul tree

**Chinmaya** (m) full of knowledge

**Chintaka** (m) philosopher

**Chintaamani** (m) the philosopher's stone

**Chintana** (m) meditation

**Chintani** (f)

**Chiraaga** (m) lamp, light

**Chiranjiva** (m) long life. Also **Chiranjeevee**. **Chiranjeeveetaa** (f) **Chiranjeevinee** (f)

**Chirantana** (m) of long standing **Chirantanee** (f)

**Chiraayu** (f) long life

**Chiti** (f) knowledge

**Chitparaa** (f) power of thinking

**Chitrabhaahu** (m) one having beautiful arms

**Chitrabhaana** (m) fire, sun

**Chitrabhanu** (m) sun

**Chitraketu** (m) one who has a beautiful banner

**Chitraaksha** (m) beautiful eyed

**Chitralekhaa** (f) an artist

**Chitrinee** (f) one endowed with many talents

**Chitraratha** (m) the sun

**Chitshakti** (f) intellectual capacity

**Chitshanti** (f) peace of mind

**Chitta** (m) knowledge

**Chittaranjana** (m) one who pleases the mind

**Chittaswarupa** (m) the supreme spirit

**Chittaprasaada** (m) happiness

**Chitvan** (m) one who meditates

**Chudaamani** (m) crest jewel

# D

**Dadhijaa** (f) a woman soft as butter

**Dadhisutaa** (f) born from the sea

**Daksha** (m) able, alert

**Dakshaa** (f) also **Dakshee** intelligent

**Dakshesha** (m) name of Shiva

**Daljita** (m) victor over the armed forces

**Dalapati** (m) commander of army

**Dama** (m) a son

**Damana** (m) taming, subduing

**Damati** (m) conquering

**Daaminee** (f) lightning

**Dandadhara** (m) one who bears the rod

**Dandin** (m) a brahmin of the fourth order

**Dariyaalaala** (m) son of the sea

**Darpaka** (m) name of Kaamadeva, god of love

**Dariyaasaaranga** (m) an expert mariner

**Darpitaa** (f) proud

**Darpinee** (f)

**Darpita** (m)

**Darshanaa** (f) one who looks beautiful

**Darshaka** (m) vision

**Darshana** (f) vision

**Darshee** (f) perceiving

**Darshitaa** (f) displayed

**Daruka** (m) the deodar tree

**Dasharatha** (m) one who has ten chariots

**Datta** (m) **Dattaa** (f) one who is given

**Dattachitta** (m) one who is engrossed in Datta

**Dayaa** (f) pity

**Dayaanidhi** (m) store of compassion, pity

**Dayaala** (m) one who has pity

**Dayaalachanda** (m) moon of mercy

**Dayaamaya** (m) full of mercy

**Dayaananda** (m) one who takes joy in being merciful

**Dayaarama** (m) Rama, the merciful

**Dayaashankara** (m) Shiva, the merciful

**Dayaavantee** (m/f) a very kind person

**Debaashish** (m) pleased by god

**Deekshaa** (f) consecration for a religious ceremony

**Deenadayaala** (m) humble, merciful

**Darpana** (m) looking glass **Darpanaa** (f)

**Dayita** (m) beloved

**Dayitaa** (f)

**Devaharshaa** (f) joy of the gods

**Dhanadaasa** (m) servant of wealth

**Dharmakirti** (m) fame of the law

**Daaruna** (m) hard, fierce

**Darvikaa** (f) a sacrificial ladle or spoon

**Dashamee** (f) the tenth day of the lunar fortnight

**Dharmalaabha** (m) profited by the law

**Dharmamitra** (m) friend of the law

**Dharmanaabha** (m) glory of Dharma

**Dharmapaala** (m) protector of the law

**Deepaka** (m) kindle

**Deepaa** (f) a shining woman

**Deepikaa** (f) one who shows the way

**Deepaalee** (f) a row of lights

**Deepakalikaa** (f) the flame of a lamp

**Deepankara** (m) one who lights the lamp

**Deepaayana** (m) pathway of a lamp

**Deependra** (m) lord of the light

**Deeptaa** (f) a lustrous woman

**Deeptaamshu** (m) the sun

**Devadaasa** (m) servant of the lord

**Devadatta** (m) gift of the god

**Devaganikaa** (f) a nymph

**Devaagni** (m) pure, holy fire

**Devajnaa** (f) a woman having knowledge of God

**Devajna** (m)

**Deva** (m) god

**Deveenaa** (f) goddess

**Devakumaara** (m) son of a god **Devakumaaree** (f)

**Devalaa** (f) female attendant of an idol

**Devaananda** (m) joy of god

**Devalataa** (f) the nava-mallikaa or double jasmine plant

**Devamayee** (f) one with god

**Devamani** (m) the jewel of Vishnu

**Devaanga** (f) a part or limb of God

**Devaanganaa** (f) a celestial damsel

**Devaamshu** (m) part of god

**Devaraaja** (m) king among gods

**Devasenaa** (f) army of gods

**Devashree** (m) fate, fortune

**Devavaanee** (f) a divine voice

**Devavrata** (m) one who has taken a religious vow

**Devendra** (m) king of gods

**Devendranaatha** (m) lord of the king of gods

**Davee** (f) goddess

**Deveebaalaa** (f) divine, godly

**Devilaala** (m) son of Devi

**Deviprasaada** (m) gift of Devi

**Devalakshmee** (f) wealth of the gods

**Devidaasa** (m) servant of the goddess

**Dhairyabaalaa** (f) endowed with courage

**Dhairyavaan**(m) one who is courageous

**Dhanada** (f) one who gifts wealth

**Dhanapati** (m) lord of wealth

**Dhanalakshmee** (f) goddess of wealth

**Dhananjaya** (m) one who wins wealth

**Dhanesha** (m) lord of wealth

**Dhanurjaya** (f) beauty of wealth

**Dharanaa** (f) the act of supporting

**Dhaneshwaree** (f) goddess of wealth

**Dhanavidyaa** (f) treasure of knowledge

**Dharaa** (f) earth

**Dhaaraa** (f) a stream of water

**Dhaarinee** (f) the earth

**Dharitree** (f) the earth

**Dharma** (m) law **Dharmaa** (f)

**Dharmajna** one who is conversant with civil and religious law

**Dharmajnaa** (f)

**Dharmadaasa** (m) servant of the law

**Dharmadeva** (m) lord of law

**Dharmamegha** (m) cloud

**Dharmayasha** (m) fame gained through religious practices

**Dharmesha** (m) master of religion

**Dharmishtaa** (f) one who has faith in religion

**Dhaatree** (f) earth

**Dhyaana** (m) meditation

**Dhyaanesha** (m) lord of mental concentration

**Dhavalaa** (f) fair complexioned

**Dipti** (f) brightness

**Dhimani** (m) one having intellect

**Dhiraaja** (m) king of the brave

**Dhiren** (m) one who is firm

**Dhirendra** (m) lord of the brave

**Dhritimaana** (m) one who is firm minded

**Divya** (m) divine

**Divyaamshu** (m) the sun

**Dhundhalee** (f) childless

**Dhrishtaketu** one whose banner is boldness

**Dhruva** (m) the polar star

**Dhrumana** (f) a firm woman

**Dhoorjati** (m) the first god

**Dhyaneshwara** (m) master of meditation

**Digambara** (m) naked

**Digambaree** (f)

**Diganta** (m) end of the horizon

**Digvijaya** (m) conquest of all directions

**Dinendra** (m) lord of the day

**Dinakara** (m) the sun

**Dishti** (f) good fortune

**Deenaa** (f) one who is in need

**Deena** (m)

**Deenaanatha** (m) lord of the needy

**Deekshaa** (f) to take a vow from 'Guru'

**Deeptaamshu** (m) ray of light

**Deepti** (f) radiant beauty

**Deeptimaana** (m) **Deeptaa** (f)

**Deepa** (m) light **Deepa** (f)

**Divaakara** (m) the sun

**Divija** (m) born in heaven

**Divyaanga** (m) divine

**Divyaanganaa** (f) a heavenly nymph

**Divyaa** (f) a radiant woman

**Divya** (m)

**Divyakaanata** (m) (kaant — husband) **Divyakaantaa** (f)

**Divyammbaree** (f) a woman who is dressed in a heavenly manner

**Divyamurti** (m) a radiant idol

**Daaruna** (m) hard, fierce

**Darvikaa** (f) a sacrificial ladle or spoon

**Dashamee** (f) the tenth day of lunar fortnight

**Dhumrikaa** (f) smoky-cheeked

**Divyendu** (m) bright moon

**Divyammbaree** (f) a woman who is dressed in a heavenly manner

**Diwaalee** (f) festival of lights

**Drashtaa** (f) a witness

**Drupada** (m) father of Draupadi

**Drashti** (f) sight

**Duhitaa** (f) daughter

**Dulaaree** (f) daughter

**Durgesha** (m) lord of Durga, Shiva

**Dwaipaayana** (m) one who lives on an island

**Dwaarkaadaas** (m) servant of Dwaraka

**Dwaarakaanaatha** (m) lord of Dwaraka

**Dwipaa** (f) female elephant

**Dwipaada** (m) with two legs

**Dwipaadee** (f)

**Dwija** (m) twice-born

**Dwirada** (m) elephant

**Dwirefa** (m) large, black bee

**Dwijaraja** (m) king of brahmins

**Dwijottama** (m) best among brahmins

**Dwivedee** (m) knowing two vedas

**Dyuti** (f) splendour

# E

**Edha** (f) prosperity
**Eil/Aila** (m) son of earth
**Ekaa** (f) alone
**Ekaagra** (m) one concentrating his attention on a fixed point
**Ekaaksha** (m) one-eyed
**Ekama** (m) unit, the figure one
**Ekataa** (m) unity
**Ekataana**(m) absorbed in thought
**Ekaatma** (m) alone
**Ekachaarinee** (f) loyal
**Ekadanta** (m) the god with one tooth or tusk
**Ekaakitaa** (f) loneliness, also **Ekaakinee** (f)
**Enakshee** (f) doe-eyed

**Ekakundala** (m) lord of the sea
**Ekalinga** (m) Shiva
**Ekanga** (m) a bodyguard
**Ekaanta** (m) solitary
**Ekaavalee** (f) string of pearls
**Ekinee** (f) one who is alone
**Ekodar** (m) born of the same womb, brother
**Ekodaraa** (f) sister
**Elaa** (f) cardamon
**Elokeshee** (f) a woman having hair like the ela creeper
**Enakshee** (f) a woman having eyes like that of a deer
**Eni** (f) a female black deer
**Esha** (m) pleasure
**Eshaa** (f) desire, wish (also **Eshanaa**)

# F/Ph

**Phalaguma** (m) producer of fruit

**Phaalgunee** (f) name of a constellation

**Falgu** (f) beautiful

**Phalana** (m) crop, fertilization

**Phalaka** (m) sky, heaven

**Phani** (m) serpent

**Phalaashaa** (f) desire for fruit of the action

**Phanishwara** (m) king of serpents

**Phaninaatha** (m) lord of serpents

**Phaneendra** (m) king of the gods

**Fatehchand** (m) success

**Phoolmaalaa** (f) garland of flowers

**Phoolmani** (f) a jewel among flowers

**Phoollaa** (f) in full bloom

**Phoollendu** (m) full moon

**Phoolrani** (f) queen of flowers

# G

**Gaathaa** (f) story written in verse

**Gaayatreenee** (f) one who sings hymns

**Gabhasti** (f) a ray, light

**Gadaadhara** (m) one who holds the club

**Gangala** (m) a precious stone

**Gagana** (m) sky, heaven

**Gaganaghosha** (m) thunder

**Gaganaviharee** (m) one who resides in the heavens

**Gahana** (m) one who has the strength of an elephant

**Gajadhara** (m) one who can handle an elephant

**Gajagaaminee** (f) one who has an elephant-like gait

**Gajaanana** (m) one who has the face of an elephant also **Gajavadana** (m)

**Gajapati** (m) lord, master

**Gajapushpee** (f) a kind of creeper

**Gajaraa** (f) wreath of flowers

**Gajendra** (m) lord of the elephants

**Gamatee** (m) jolly, gay

**Gambheera** (m) serious, considerate

**Gambheeraa** (f)

**Ganadhara** (m) chief of a group

**Ganaka** (m) an astrologer

**Ganakee** or **Ganikaa** (f)

**Gananaatha** (m) group, clan

**Ganaraaja** (m) lord of the clan

**Gandharva** (m) a celestial musician

**Ghandharvee** (f)

**Gandhaakshata** (m) sandalwood paste and rice used in worship

**Gandhaa** (f) a sweet smelling woman also **Gandhalee**

**Gandhamadana** (m) a large black bee

**Gandhaharikaa** (f) a person who prepares perfumes

**Gandhavatee** (f) the earth, wine

**Gandhalataa** (f) the priyangu creeper

**Gangadatta** (m) gift of the Gangas

**Gangaadhara** (m) Shiva

**Gangodaka** (m) water of Ganges

**Gangotree** (f) origin of the Ganges

**Gambhira** (m) dignified

**Gambhiraa** (f)

**Ganasaagara** (m) ocean of virtue

**Gandhaali** (f) perfumed

**Gaveshanaa** (f) search

**Gulikaa** (f) a ball, a pearl

**Gunakara** (m) treasure of virtues

**Garuda** (m) the king of birds

**Garimaa** (f) greatness

**Garjana** (m) loud cry

**Gati** (f) speed

**Gauraanga** (m) fair complexioned

**Guaraanganaa** (f)

**Gaandhaara** (m) third note on the Indian musical scale

**Gaurava** (m) pride, respect

**Gavana** (f) upper garment or sari, worn by women

**Gaveshaka** (m) researcher

**Gayan** (m) sky

**Gayand** (m) elephant

**Gehini** (f) housewife

**Geeta** (m) a song **Geeti** (f)

**Geetaa** (f) the lord's song

**Geetikaa** (f) a short song

**Ghanashyaama** (m) black as a cloud

**Ghritaachi** (f) night

**Dhataakarna** (m) one who has ears like a bell

**Ghantaali** (f) a string of small bells

**Ghataja** (m) born from a pot

**Ghanvallikaa** (f) a creeper of clouds

**Gunidatta** (m) given by a virtuous man

**Ghatikaa** (f) a small water jar used to measure time

**Ghoshanaa** (f) declaration

**Ghughari** (f) bracelet with jingling bells

**Giraa** (f) speech

**Giri** (m) mountain

**Giribaalaa** (f) daughter of the mountain

**Girilala** (m) son of the mountain

**Giridhara** (m) one who holds up the mountain

**Girvaana** (m) language of gods

**Grishmaa** (f) summer

**Girijaa** (f) daughter of the mountain

**Girijaapati** (m) lord or husband of Girijaa. Also **Girijaavallabha, Girijaavara** and **Girijaanatha**

**Girijaasuta** (m) son of Girijaa

**Girijaaprasaada** (m) Girijaa's blessings

**Girijatanayaa** (f) daughter of Girijaa

**Giriraja** (m) king of mountains

**Gitaanjali** (f) handful of poems or songs

**Geetasudha** (f) sweet music

**Gobinda** (m) cowherd

**Gokarna** (m) a cow's ear

**Gokula** (m) herd of cows

**Golakhnaatha** (m) master of the globe

**Gomateshwara** (m) a kind of gem

**Gomukha** (m) mouth of a cow

**Gopaa** (f) cowherd

**Gopaala** (m)

**Gopee** (f) milkmaid

**Gopabaalaa** (f) daughter of a cowherd

**Gopaladaasa** (m) servant of Gopaala

**Gopaalee** (f) woman belonging to the tribe of cow herds. Also **Gopaalikaa**

**Gopana** (m) protection

**Gopanaa** (f)

**Goptaa** (m) guardian

**Gorakhanaatha** (m) one who has control over his senses

**Gorala** (m/f) likeable

**Gorambh** (m) sky with dark clouds

**Goraande** (f) fair complexioned

**Gormaa** (f) Gauri

**Goshaalaka** (m) master of the cow stable

**Goshpa** (m) step of a cow

**Goshti** (f) conversation

**Goteeta** (m) one that is beyond cognition of the senses

**Govinda** (m) keeper of cows

**Grahesha** (m) lord of the planets

**Granthika** (m) astrologer

**Grathal** (m) amazement

**Gruheet** (m) that which is understood

**Gulaaba** (m/f) rose

**Gulaabee** (f) rosy, pleasing

**Gulaal** (m/f) slightly fragrant reddish powder

**Gunaadhya** (m) rich in virtues

**Gunadhara** (m) one who has character

**Gunaakara** (m) endowed with all virtues

**Gunavatee** (f) a virtuous woman

**Gunaratna** (m) a jewel of virtue

**Gunasundari** (f) the supreme being

**Gunfanaa** (f) one whose life is woven of virtues

**Gunajana** (m) one who knows how to admire virtues

**Gunanidhi** (m) a treasure-house of virtues

**Guniyal** (f) a virtuous woman

**Gunee** (m) one who is virtuous

**Gunjaa** (f) small plant with red and black berries

**Gunjaka** (m) resonance

**Gurbachan** (m) **Guruvachana** the promise of the guru

**Gurudeepa** (m) lamp of the guru

**Gurudayaala** (m) the compassionate guru

**Guru** (m) teacher, master, priest

**Gurucharana** (m) at the feet of the guru

**Gurumeet** (m) friend of the guru

**Gurunaama** (m) name of the guru

**Gurumukha** (m) in the image of the guru

**Gursharana** (m) one who has come to the guru for refuge

**Gurudaasa** (m) servant of the guru

**Gurudatta** (m) gift of the guru

# H

Haalaa (f) wine

Hamsa (m) swan Hansi (f)

Hamsamaalaa (f) a flight of swans

Hamsanandinee (f) with slender waist

Hamsaraaja (m) king of swans

Hansikaa (f) little swan

Harini/Harinee (f) doe

Harshana (m) pleasant

Harshini (f)

Harshaveena (f) a musical instrument

Hemaketaki (f) the ketaki plant

Hemanti (f) relating to the Hemanta season

Hemavarnaa (f) golden complexioned

Hara (m) Shiva

Harabaalaa (f) daughter of Hara

Harashekhar (m) Hara's crest

Harasiddha (m) eternal Shiva

Haaraavali (f) garland of pearls

Haardikaa (f) affectionate

Haren (m) great Shiva

Hari (m) Vishnu, the sun

Haribaalaa (f) daughter of Hari

Harbansa (m) belonging to the family of Hari

Harivamsha (m) name of purana

Haribhakti (m) devotion to Hari

Harichandana (m) a kind of yellow paste

Haricharana (m) at the feet of the lord

Haridaasa (m) servant of Hari

Harihara (m) Shiva and Vishnu together

Harikaanta (m) dear to the lord

Haradeva (m) Shiva

Haradevee (f) Paarvatee

Harilala (m) son of Hari

Harimani (f) jewel

Haramedhas (m) sacrifice

Harivallabha (m) dear of Hari

Harindra (m) lord Hari, also Harindranaatha

Harinaakshee (f) doe-eyed

Harinivas (m) house of Hari

Hari Om (m) name of Brahma

Haripaala (m) one who protects Hari, lion

Hariprapada (m) blessings of Hari

Haripriyaa (f) beloved of Hari

Hariraaja (m) king of lions

Harismita (m) smile of Hari

Halaayudha (m) one who carries the plough as his weapon

Harivadana (m) possessing a face like Hari

Harivatsa (m) name of Arjuna

Harivilaasa (m) pleasure of Hari

Harsha (m) joy, delight

Harshaa (f)

Harshula (m) a deer

**Harshada** (m) giver of pleasure
**Harshadaa** (f) also **Harshidaa**
**Harshala** (m) a lover
**Harshanaa** (f) one who causes delight
**Harshinee** (f) a woman in joyful mood
**Harshaveena** (f) a musical instrument
**Harshavardhana** (m) one who increases joy
**Harshumatee** (f) one filled with joy
**Hasikaa** (f) laughter
**Hasmukha** (m) one having a smiling face **Hasumatee** (f)
**Hastinee** (f) elephant
**Hastin** (m) one who has hands
**Haatakeshwara** (m) lord of gold
**Havirdhaama** (m) a place of sacrifice
**Hayagriva** (m) one having the head of a horse
**Hima** (f) a mass of snow
**Heenaa** (f) a fragrance
**Heeraka** (m) a diamond
**Hemaa** (f) golden
**Hemachandra** (m) golden moon
**Hemaadri** (m) mountain of gold
**Hemadaasa** (m) slave of gold
**Hemaanga** (m) one having a shining body
**Hemaangee** (f)
**Hemamaalini** (f) garland of gold
**Hemantee** (f) one who shines like gold
**Hemavatee** (f) bright as gold
**Hemendra** (m) lord of gold
**Hemaraaja** (m) king of gold

**Hemavateenandana** (m) son of Hemavatee
**Hemalataa** (f) golden creeper
**Hemila** (f) golden flower
**Heramba** (m) boastful
**Himachala** (m) unmoving
**Himajaa** (f) born of Paarvatee
**Himaadrivadana** (m) serene
**Himarashmi** (m) moon with rays as cold as snow
**Himasutaa** (f) daughter of the snows
**Himaavata** (m) mountain king
**Heeraa** (m/f) diamond
**Heeraalakshmee** (f) beautiful as a diamond
**Heeraachanda** (m) diamond-like moon
**Heeraamana** (m) a diamond-sharp mind
**Hiranya** (m) wealth
**Hiranyadaa** (f) giver of wealth
**Hiranyaaksha** (m) one having golden eyes
**Hiranyamaya** (m) golden
**Hiranyamayee** (f)
**Hiranyeretas** (m) name of Shiva
**Hiresha** (m) king of gems
**Hitaarthee** (f) one who does good to others
**Holikaa** (f) sister of Hiranya-kashyapa (a festival)
**Hree** (f) to blush with modesty
**Hridaya** (m) the heart
**Hridayanatha** (m) beloved
**Hridayasudhaa** (f) nectar of the heart
**Hridayesha** (m) lord of the heart **Hridayeshaa** (f)
**Hrishikesha** (m) one who controls the senses
**Hridayeshwara** (m) husband

26

**Ibhi** (f) an elephant
**Ibhaanana** (m) elephant faced
**Idaa** (f) speech, earth
**Ilaa** (f) praise
**Idaavidaa** (f) a scholar in speech
**Idhma** (m) fuel
**Idhajivha** (m) one who carries fuel
**Ihaa** (f) wish, desire
**Ijyaa** (f) sacrifice
**Ikshaa** (f) sight
**Ikshitaa** (f) what is seen
**Ikshulaa** (f) name of a river
**Ikshu** (m) sugarcane
**Ikshumaalinee** (f) a florist
**Ikshumatee** (f) one who possesses sugarcane
**Ilesha** (m) lord of the earth
**Ileshaa** (f)
**Ilikaa** (f) earth
**Ikshikaa** (f) a glance
**Indaalee** (f) to become powerful
**Indumauli** (m) the moon-created god
**Indeevara** (m) the blue lotus
**Indra** (m) the god of rain
**Indrabaalaa** (f) daughter of Indra
**Indrabha** (m) light of Indra
**Indradatta** (m) gift of Indra
**Indrabhattaarika** (f) venerable
**Indradyumna** (m) splendour of Indra

**Indrajit** (m) conqueror of Indra
**Indrakeela** (m) banner of Indra
**Indraakshee** (f) beautiful-eyed
**Indraanee** (f) wife of Indra
**Indraneela** (m) an emerald
**Indraajuna** (m) bright Indra
**Indravaaha** (m) Indra's horse
**Indravadana** (m) one who has the face of Indra
**Indumatee** (f) full moon
**Indu** (m/f) moon
**Indujaa** (f) daughter of the moon
**Indukaanta** (m) handsome as the moon
**Indukalaa** (f) like the moon
**Inesha** (m) king of kings
**Ipsit** (f) desire **Ipsitaa** (f)
**Iraa** (f) the earth
**Iresha** (m) lord of the earth
**Irikaa** (f) also **Illikaa** little earth
**Irmaa** (m) the sun
**Isha** (m) ruler, master
**Ishaana** (m) the sun
**Ishaanee** (f) Durgaa
**Irshikaa** (f) a painter's brush
**Ishita** (m) one who desires to rule **Ishitaa** (f) greatness
**Iishm** (m) the season of spring
**Ishwara** (m) powerful, the supreme god
**Ishwarakaantaa** (f) name of Durgaa

# J

**Jagata** (m) world
**Jagadambaa** (f) mother of the world
**Jagadeva/Jagadisha** (m) lord of the world
**Jagadeepa** (m) light of the world
**Jagajeeta** (m) conqueror of the world
**Jagajeevana** (m) life of the world
**Jagmi** (m) wind
**Jagannaatha** (m) lord of the universe
**Jaganu** (m) fire
**Jaganmohan** (m) one who attracts the world
**Jagatee** (f) the earth
**Jaagruti** (f) awakening also **Jagaritaa** (f)
**Janikaa** (f) one who give birth to
**Jananee** (f) a mother
**Jaya** (m) victory
**Jayadeepa** (m) light of victory
**Jayadeva/Jaideva** (m) god of victory
**Jayaadevee** (f) goddess of victory
**Jayaraaja** (m) victorious king
**Jayasukha** (m) success, happiness
**Jalabaalaa** (f) child of the water
**Jalabaalikaa** (f) lightning
**Jaladhara** (m) cloud
**Jaladhaaraa** (f) stream of water

**Jalaadhi** (m) ocean
**Jalajaa** (f) lotus
**Jalajaakshi** (f) lotus-eyed
**Jaalandharaa** (f) a net, web
**Jalaarka** (m) the image of the sun reflected in water
**Jalaarnava** (m) rainy season
**Jalasandha**(m) sandh union
**Jalini** (f) one who lives in water
**Jalaneeli** (f) moss
**Jamadagni** (m) fire-eater
**Jayapaala/Jaipaala** (m) one who protects success
**Jamunaa** (f) name of a river
**Jamanaadaas** (m) servant of Jamuna
**Jamanaalaala** (m) son of Jamuna
**Janaardana** (m) one who helps people
**Janamitra** (m) friend of the people
**Janesha** (m) master of all
**Jany** (m) fire, living being
**Jataadhara** (m) knotted hair
**Jataashankara** (m) matted hair
**Jataayu** (m) a semi-divine bird
**Jasaraaja** (m) king of fame
**Jasveer** (m) hero of fame
**Jaswant** (m) victorious
**Jaswantee** (f) a woman of great renown
**Jawaahara** (m) jewel
**Jayaditya** (m) victorious sun
**Jayakaanta** (m) pleasing success
**Jeevana** (m) life

**Jayashekhara** (m) crest of victory

**Jayaswaminee** (f) goddess of victory

**Jayajaa/Jayin** (m) one who is victorious

**Jayeetaa** (f) a successful woman

**Jitendra** (m) lord of conquerors

**Jeevanadaasa** (m) servant of life

**Jeevanteeka** (f) a flower

**Jharnaa** (f) brook

**Jhashaanka** (m) uncontrolled

**Jhasha** (m) heat, warmth

**Jhaanavikaa** (f) name of Ganges

**Jhankaarinee** (f) murmur

**Jatila** (m) lion **Jatilaa** (f)

**Jidvisha** (m) visha    poison

**Jigisha** (m) one who desires to conquer **Jigishaa** (f)

**Jignyassu** (m) one who thirsts for knowledge

**Jinabhadra** (m) bhadra happy, good

**Jinendra** (m) lord of life

**Jishnu** (m) triumphant

**Jitavrata** (m) one who has kept his vow

**Jivaraaia** (m) lord of life

**Jivyaa** (f) means of livelihood

**Jnapti** (f) intelligence

**Jnaanadeepa** (m) light of knowledge

**Jnaanaagni** (m) knowledge as illuminating as fire

**Jnaanadhan** (m) wealth of knowledge

**Jnaaneshwara** (m) the wisest

**Jnyaana** (m) understanding

**Jnaanamaya** (m) full of knowledge

**Jnyanamurti** (m) one who is the embodiment of knowledge

**Jnyaapaka** (m) a teacher

**Jnyaanaprakaasha** (m) light of knowledge

**Jneya** (m) god

**Jyoti** (f) flame, brightness

**Jyotikaa** (f) a kind of flower

**Jyotindra** (m) lord of light

**Jyotsanaa** (f) moonlight

**Jyotsanaalataa** (f) moonlight creeper

**Jwaalaa** (f) flame

**Jwalanta** (m) shining

**Jugalakishora** (m) jugal    a pair, kishora    child

**Jyeshtlaa** (f) eldest sister

**Jnanadaa** (f) one who gives supreme knowledge

**Jnanemaya** (m) full of wisdom **Gnyanamayi** (f)

**Jyotirmaya** (m) starry

**Jyotishmati** (f) luminous

# K

Kadamba (m) name of a tree
Kaadambaree (f) cuckoo
Ka (m) the lord of creatures (pronoun : who)
Kaahini (f) a young woman
Kairava (m) white lotus, also, a cheat
Kairvinee (f) lotus plant bearing white lotuses
Kairavee (f) moonlight
Kaishika (m) as thin as hair
Kaajala (f) kohl
Kaakalee (f) tender, sweet tone
Kakudmi (m) a mountain
Kalaachanda (m) a small part of the moon
Kaaleekaa (f) group of dark clouds
Kaalanjaya (m) one who has conquered time
Kalaapee (m) peacock
kalaavatee (f) the embodiment of art
Kalahmasa (m) swan
Kalahamsee (f)
Kaalee (f) form of power
Kalila (m) mixed, deep
Kaaleecharana (m) at the feet of goddess Kaalee
Kalinda (m) sun
Kalinga (m) a bird
Kaalingi (f) a woman from Kaling
Kalita (m) known, understood
Kallola (m) joy
Kallolee (f) one who enjoys
Kalpkataa (f) imagination

Kallolinee (f) one who is always happy
Kalpa (m) determination
Kalpalataa (f) lataa  creeper kalpa  secret wish
Kalpanaa (f) imagination
Kalpan (m)
Kaalkaa (f) deep
Kallee (f) an ornament worn on the wrist
Kalyaana (m) blessed
Kalyaanee (f) fortunate
Kalyaanadaasa (m) servant of prosperity
Kaamadeva (m) god of love
Kaamaakshee (f) one with voluptuous eyes
Kamala (m/f) lotus
Kamalaa (f) an excellent woman
Kamalaakara (m) a lake full of lotuses
Kaamarekhaa (f) literally, line of love
Kaamalataa (f) creeper of love
Kamalesha (m) lord of the lotus
Kamalaakshee (f) lotus-eyed
Kaamalee (f) one full of desire
Kamalakanta (m) lord of the lotus
Kalpaka (m) a rite
Kamalinee (f) a lotus plant
Kaivalya (m) perfect isolation
Kailaasnaatha (m) lord of Kailas
Kaaminee (f) full of desire

**Kaameshwara** (m) one having full control over passion
**Kaameshwaree** (f)
**Kamalanayana** (m) lotus-eyed
**Kamalanayanaa** (f)
**Kaamaayudha** (m) cupid's arrow
**Kanakamudraa** (f) a gold ring
**Kanakvi** (f) a small kite
**Kanakvaa** (m)
**Kaanam** (m/f) earth with black soil
**Kaanana** (f) forest
**Kaanchana** (m) gold
**Kaanchangauree** (f) fair complexioned
**Kanchanlaala** (m) son of gold
**Kaanchee** (f) waistband with bells
**Kandarpa** (m) god of love
**Kandarpabaalaa** (f) daughter of cupid
**Kadali** (f) the banana tree
**Kangana** (f) a type of bangle
**Kanikaa** (f) an atom
**Kankana** (f) a tinkling ornament
**Kanja** (m) Brahma, lotus
**Kanjaka** (m) a bird
**Kanjana** (m) god of love
**Kanajara** (m) an elephant
**Kanjaree** (f) a musical instrument
**Kaanajee** (m) Krishna
**Kanka** (m) crane, heron
**Kaankshaa** (f) wish
**Kaankshinee** (f) one who wishes
**Kaanta** (m) lovely, beautiful
**Kaantaa** (f) beloved
**Kaanti** (m/f) lustre
**Kanwala** (f) lotus
**Kanyaa** (f) daughter

**Kanwalajeet** (m) jeet victory
**Kapardi** (m) Shiva
**Kapardinee** (f) Paarvatee
**Kapardikaa** (f) a small shell
**Kapidhwaja** (m) kapi monkey, dhwaj flag
**Kapinjala** (m) partridge
**Kapinjalaa** (f) a river
**Kanaka** (f) gold, wealth
**Kanakalataa** (f) a creeper
**Kaanchana** (f) gold
**Kaantidaa** (f) one who gives light
**Kadambini** (f) garland of clouds
**Kalhaara** (m) water lily
**Kallola** (m) joy, happiness
**Kallolini** (f) surging stream
**Kalpikaa** (f) fit, proper
**Kalpitaa** (f) formed, arranged
**Kanakaprabhaa** (f) splendour of gold
**Kanakasundari** (f) beautiful as gold
**Karnikaa** (f) kind of creeper
**Karana** (m) reason
**Karaandeep** (m) light of action
**Karanee** (f) action, miracle
**Karena** (m) name of a flower
**Kaarikaa** (f) actress, dancer
**Karikrishna** (m) black elephant
**Karini** (f) elephant
**Kautuki** (f) full of curiosity
**Kavana** (m) water
**Karmashreshtha** (m) one who is great in action
**Karna** (m) literally, ear
**Karnadhaara** (m) leader
**Karnaka** (m) auricle of the heart
**Karnikaa** (f) bud

**Karpoora** (m) camphor
**Karpooree** (f)
**Karpurgauraa** (f) Paarvatee
**Karpurigaur** (m) Shiva
**Kaartikeya** (m) the god of war
**Kaarti** (m) name of a month
**Karunaa** (f) compassion
**Karunaanidhi** (m) treasure of pity
**Kaasu** (f) light, lustre
**Kaasheeaa** (m) name of a bird
**Kaasheeraama** (m) one who pleases Kaashi
**Kaashtaa** (f) direction
**Kaashya** (m) a kind of grass
**Kaashyapa** (m) tortoise
**Kaashyapee** (f) earth
**Kastura** (f) musk
**Kasturee** (f)
**Kastureekaa** (f) rut of a deer
**Khadirikaa** (f) the moon
**Kathaa** (m) story
**Kathaarnava** (m) sea of stories
**Kaatyaayinee** (f) Paarvatee
**Kaumudi** (f) moonlight
**Kausara** (m) a pool in heaven
**Kausha** (m) silken
**Kaushala** (m) clever, skilled
**Kaushika** (m) sentiment of love
**Kaushikaa** (f) a cup
**Kaustubha** (m) a precious stone
**Kaavalee** (f) bangle
**Kaaveree** (f) a courtesan
**Kavi** (m) a wise man
**Kavitaa** (f) poetry
**Karmashreshtha** (m) one who is great in actions
**Keera** (m) parrot
**Keertana** (m) song of praise

**Kekaa** (f) cry of a peacock
**Kekaavalee** (f) a chorus of peacock cries
**Kesaree** (m/f) saffron
**Kesari** (m) saffron coloured
**Keshava** (m) having curly hair
**Keshavananda** (m) one who has supreme bliss in the lord
**Keshina** (m) lion
**Keshinee** (f) braid of hair
**Keshinivadana** (m) destroyer of Keshin
**Ketaka** (m) kind of fragrant shrub
**Ketakee** (f) agave
**Ketana** (m) sign, mark
**Kevala** (m) pure
**Keyura** (m) an amulet
**Keyuree** (f) one wearing a bracelet
**Khagaadhiraaja** (m) lord of the birds
**Khandinee** (f) earth
**Khagendra** (m) lord of the birds
**Khadyot** (m) glow worm
**Khanjana** (m/f) dimple
**Khelaiyo** (m) a sportsman
**Khelani** (f) a doll
**Khushaal** (m) happy, healthy
**Khushaali** (f)
**Khushilal/Khushiram** (m) happy
**Khushee** (f) pleasure
**Khushamana** (m) one with a happy mind
**Khushawanta** (m) one endowed with happiness
**Khyaati** (f) fame
**Kim** (m) a bird
**Kinjala** (f) brook
**Kinkanee** (f) waistband with small bells

32

**Kinnara** (m) a demi-god
**Kinnaree** (f)
**Kirana** (m/f) ray
**Kiranmayee** (f) full of rays
**Kashyapee** (m) earth
**Khagesha** (m) the eagle
**Kinjalka** (f) flower pollen
**Komala** (m) tender
**Komalaa** (f)
**Kshemalataa** (f) a creeper of welfare
**Kumaarila** (m) a learned person
**Kiraata** (m) hunter
**Kiraati** (f) Paarvatee
**Kireeta** (m) crown
**Kireeti** (m) one who wears a crown
**Kirtana/Keertan** (m) song of praise
**Keertaniya** (m) one worthy of praise
**Kirtaara** (m) the creator
**Keerti** (m) fame, glory
**Keertidaa** (f) one who bestows fame
**Keertideva** (m) god of fame
**Keertikumaara** (m) prince of fame
**Keertimanta** (m) one who enjoys glory
**Kripaa** (m/f) mercy, favour
**Kripaashankara** (m) one who bestows favours
**Kishoree** (f) a young girl
**Kishora** (m) youthful colt
**Kohinoor** (m) mountain of light
**Kokila** (m) cuckoo **Kokilaa** (f)
**Komala** (f) tender
**Komalaangee** (f) one who has a tender body

**Kraanti** (f) revolution
**Kratu** (m) talent, power
**Krishna** (m) literally 'black'
**Krishnaa** (f) name of a river
**Kirti** (f) action
**Krishnaamukha** (m) one who has the face of Krishna
**Krishnavallee** (f) black tulsi
**Krishnee** (f) a dark night
**Kritaanta** (m) god of death
**Kriyaa** (f) performance
**Krushnee** (f) dark night
**Krutamaalaa** (f) one wearing a garland
**Kshaa** (f) earth that is cultivated
**Kshamaa** (f) forgiveness
**Kshaantee** (f) tolerance
**Kshapaa** (f) night
**Kshapaachara** (m) one who wanders at night
**Kshapaakara** (m) the moon
**Kshapaanaatha** (m) lord of the night
**Kshapaapati** (m) husband of the night
**Kshapendra** (m) king of the night
**Kshemaa** (f) prosperous
**Kshemendra** (m) lord of welfare
**Kubera** (m) god of riches
**Kshipraa** (f) fast
**Kshiti** (f) the earth
**Kshitija** (m) horizon
**Kshitinaatha** (m) lord of the earth
**Kshitipaala** (m) king
**Kshiteesh** (m) lord of the world
**Kshoni** (f) earth
**Kshmaapati** (m) the king

**Kulaanganaa** (f) a woman from a good, noble family

**Kulapati** (m) the head of a family

**Kulabhooshana** (m) one who brings honour and glory to the family

**Kuladeepa** (m) also **Kuldip** one who is the light of the family

**Kulika** (m) of a good family

**Kulina** (m) of noble birth

**Kumaara** (m) young boy

**Kumaaree** (f) damsel

**Kumuda** (f) a white lotus which blooms only at night

**Kumudachandra** (m) lotus of the moon

**Kumudini** (f) a water lily

**Kumudasundari** (f) beautiful as the lotus

**Kumudvatee** (f) the lotus plant

**Kundana** (m) pure gold

**Kundanikaa** (f) a jasmine creeper

**Kundanagauree** (f) golden-white complexion

**Kunja** (f) grove of trees

**Kunjala** (f) koel

**Ketan** (m) a dwelling

**Kusumachandara** (m) saffron, outward affection

**Kunjalataa** (f) creeper in a grove

**Kuntala** (m/f) lock of hair

**Kuntalaa** (f) one with long hair

**Kuntesha** (m) master of spears

**Kunwar** (m) prince

**Kurangee** (f) doe **Kuranga** (m)

**Kushaadaa** (m/f) straight-forward

**Kushala** (m) healthy, happy

**Kushilava** (m) bard, singer

**Kustubha** (m) the ocean

**Kusuma** (f) flower, blossom

**Kusumaakara** (m) garden

**Kusumaayudha** (m) one whose weapon is a flower

**Kusumachandara** (m) moon flower

**Kusumita** (m/f) filled with flowers

**Kovida** (m) learned, wise

34

# L

**Laabha** (m) profit
**Laghimaa** (f) lightness
**Lajjaa** (f) bashfulness
**Lajjeetaa** (f) a bashful woman
**Lajjaasheela** (f) a modest
woman
**Laajawanti** (f) one who is
modest and bashful
**Lakshana** (f) symbol
**Lakshitaa** (f) noticeable
**Lakshmana** (m) prosperous
**Lakshmee** (f) goddess of
beauty and prosperity
**Lalanaa** (f) a woman
**Lalanikaa** (f) caress
**Lalita** (m) **Lalitaa** (f) playful
**Laalasaa** (f) ardent desire
**Lalitachandra** (m) beautiful
moon
**Lalitaaditya** (m) beautiful sun
**Lalitamohana** (m) beautiful
and attractive
**Lalitaanga** (m) one with a
beautiful body
**Lalitaangee** (f)
**Lankaa** (f) unchaste
**Lankaadhipa** (m) lord of
Lankaa
**Lasikaa** (f) dancer
**Lataa** (f) creeper
**Lataamani** (f) jewel

**Lataakara** (m) a mass of
creepers
**Latakastureekaa** (f) musk
creeper
**Latikaa** (f) a small creeper
**Lavanaa** (m) lustre, beauty
**Lavangalataa** (f) a creeper of
cloves
**Lavangee** (f) the clove plant
**Laavanyaprabhaa** (f) light of
beauty
**Laavanyamayi** (f) one endowed
with beauty and charm
**Leelaa** (f) charming
**Lekhaa** (f) a line, lightning
**Leelaadhara** (m) name of
Vishnu
**Lochanaa** (f) one with
beautiful eyes
**Lotikaa** (f) one who is tearful
**Lokaadhipa** (m) lord of the
world. Also, **Lokaadheesha,
Lokanaatha, Lokesha,
Lokapati**
**Lokaprakasha** (m) light of the
world
**Lomaa** (f) one with long hair
**Lomaharshana** (m) one who
thrills
**Lolitaa** (f) one who is roving
**Lopaa** (f) loss

35

# M

**Maadhabee** (f) honey-like sweet

**Maadhava** (m) husband of Lakshmi

**Maadhavee** (f) a name of Lakshmi

**Maadhuree** (f) a sweet woman

**Maadhuramohana** (m) Krishna the handsome

**Maalaa** (f) a garland

**Maalatee** (f) a virgin

**Maalaavati** (f) name of a river

**Maalaashree** (f) beautiful garland

**Maalikaa** (f) a necklace

**Maalin** (m) one wearing a garland

**Maalinee** (f) a florist

**Maanika** (f) ruby

**Maardava** (m) softness

**Maartanda** (m) the sun

**Maatanga** (m) an elephant

**Maatangee** (f) Paarvatee

**Maayaa** (f) illusion

**Madana** (m) Cupid, god of love

**Madanaa** (f) goddess of love, Rati

**Madanaa** (m) intoxicating

**Madani** (f)

**Madanamohinee** (f) an attractive woman who rouses passion

**Madanamanjushaa** (f) a casket of love

**Madanalalitaa** (f) a woman made beautiful by love

**Madanashalakaa** (f) cuckoo

**Madayantikaa** (f) a variety of jasmine

**Madhu** (m) nectar, honey

**Madhubaalaa** (f) young and sweet

**Madhulikaa** (f) sweet like honey

**Madhujaa** (f) earth

**Madhukaanta** (m) a pleasing husband

**Madhukaantaa** (f)

**Madhukara** (m) bee, lover

**Madhukaarikaa** (f) a large, black bee

**Madhulikaa** (f) pollen, black mustard

**Madhumaalaa** (f) a beautiful garland

**Madhumanjaree** (f) a beautiful sprout

**Madhumatee** (f) a sweet-tempered woman

**Madhumeetaa** (f) a moderate, sweet woman

**Madhupa** (m) one who drinks honey

**Madhupadma** (m) sweet-scented lotus

**Madhupreetaa** (f) one fond of honey

**Madhuraa** (f) melodious

**Madhuraka** (m) charming

**Madhuraakshee** (f) one with beautiful eyes

**Maadhurya** (f) sweetness

**Madhurimaa** (f) beauty

**Madhureetaa** (f) sweetness

**Madhusakha** (m) god of love

**Madadhumadhvi** (f) a kind of intoxicating drink

**Madhushree** (f) a delightful beauty

**Madhusudana** (m) sudan to kill

**Madhuyaaminee** (f) sweet night

**Madiraa** (f) goddess of wine

**Madiraksha** (m) one who has eyes as red as madiraa

**Madiraakshee** (f)

**Madirekshana** (f) one having intoxicating eyes

**Madhurasaa** (f) a bunch of grapes

**Mahaabaahu** (m) powerful

**Mahaabali** (m) very strong

**Mahaadeva** (m) the most powerful god

**Mahaadevee** (f)

**Manotosh** (m) satisfaction of the king

**Mahaananda** (m) the great bliss of final beatitude

**Maheepati** (m) the king

**Mahaashuklaa** (f) extreme whiteness

**Mahaaprabhaa** (f) one of extreme splendour

**Mahaavidyaa** (f) great knowledge

**Mahaaveera** (m) most courageous among men

**Mahendra** (m) name of Indra

**Mahesha** (m) name of Shiva

**Maheshanee** (f) Paarvatee

**Maharshi** (m) a great sage

**Maheshwaree** (f) Durgaa

**Mainaakee** (f) Paarvatee

**Maitreya** (m) friend

**Maitreyee** (f)

**Makaranda** (m) the bee

**Malaya** (m) the garden of Indra

**Malayagiri** (m) the Malaya mountain

**Manana** (m) meditation

**Manaalee** (f) a friend of the mind

**Maanasa** (m) born from the mind

**Manasvinee** (f) a wise or virtuous woman

**Maanavatee** (f) a high-spirited woman

**Mandaara** (m) flower

**Mandaakinee** (f) Gangaa

**Manobhirama** (m) one with a pleasing mind

**Manaskaanta** (m) dear to the mind

**Manaprasaada** (m) one who is mentally calm

**Manoranjana** (m) one who pleases the mind

**Manohara** (m) one who wins over the mind

**Maanavendra** (m) king among men

**Mohita** (m) one who is ensnared in illusion

**Mohitaa** (f)

**Manjaa** (f) a cluster of blossoms

**Manjikaa** (f) a courtesan

**Mandiraa** (f) a dwelling

**Manendra** (m) king of the mind

**Mangala** (m) prosperous

**Mangalaa** (f)

**Manahaara** (m) a charmer

**Mani** (m/f) gem, precious stone

**Manibhadra** (m) secure as a jewel

**Manidhara** (m) one who wears a jewel

**Manikantha** (m) the blue jay

**Manimaalaa** (f) a necklace of jewels

**Maanika** (m/f) a ruby

**Manikaa** (f) jewel, gem

**Manilaala** (m) a jewel of a son

**Maaninee** (f) a strong-minded, proud woman

**Maniraama** (m) a jewel of a man

**Manishankara** (m) Shiva

**Manishaa** (f) wisdom, intelligence

**Manishi** (m) wise, learned

**Manishina** (m) an intelligent man

**Manishikaa** (f) mind's desire

**Manjaree** (f) sprout, spring

**Manjarikaa** (f) small flower bud

**Manindra** (m) diamond

**Manjughoshaa** (f) one who receives a guest with sweet acclamation

**Manjukeshee** (f) one with beautiful hair

**Manjulaa** (f) lovely, beautiful

**Manjula** (m) handsome

**Manjulakshmee** (f) queen of beauty

**Manjushaa** (f) a trunk or box

**Mamataa** (f) love

**Manmatha** (m) god of love

**Manobhaava** (m) one who exists in the mind

**Manojna** (m) one who is attractive

**Manoja** (m) born of the mind

**Manoramaa** (f) beautiful

**Manoratha** (m) desire, wish

**Manorathaa** (f)

**Mantranaa** (f) consultation

**Manoritaa** (f) beauty

**Mandaa** (f) one who is slow

**Manasukha** (m) happiness of the mind

**Manatosha** (m) total satisfaction of the mind

**Manu** (m) to think

**Marut** (m) wind

**Marutapati** (m) king of the winds

**Maatraa** (f) a moment, wealth

**Maraala** (m/f) swan

**Maraali** (f)

**Maraalikaa** (f) small swan

**Mareechi** (m) ray of light

**Matsyendra** (m) king of fishes

**Matsyagandhaa** (f) one who smells like fish

**Maulika** (m) original

**Maulikaa** (f)

**Maulina** (m) original, best

**Maayaa** (f) an illusory image

**Mayanaa** (f) Paarvatee

**Mayanka** (m) moon

**Mayukha** (m) peacock

**Mayuree** (f) peahen

**Mayura** (m) peacock

**Mayuraa/Mayurikaa** (f) peahen

**Maayuraaja** (m) maayu sun

**Medhaa** (f) victorious through the intellect **Medhaaji** (m)

**Medhaarthee** (f) wise

**Medhas** (m) retentive faculty

**Medhaavan** (m) one who is wise **Medhaavini** (f)

**Medhikaa** (f) the henna bush

**Medinee** (f) earth

**Meenaa** (f) fish

**Meghabhooti** (m) lightning

**Meenakshee** (f) one who is fish-eyed

**Meghamaalaa** (f) garland of clouds

**Meeraa** one who is circumscribed

**Meghanaada** (m) thunder

**Meghadatta** (m) gift of the clouds

**Megharanjani** (f) glory of the clouds

**Meghasandhi** (m) union with clouds

**Meghashyaama** (m) black like a cloud

**Meghavarna** (m) dark as a cloud

**Mehaa** (f) rain

**Mehula** (m) rain **Mehulaa** (f)

**Mihikaa** (f) dew, mist

**Mihir** (m) the sun

**Milind** (m) honey bee

**Milon** (m) **Milana/Milonee** (f) meeting, getting together

**Miraata** (f) mirror

**Mitesha** (m) one with few desires

**Mithila** (m) area, kingdom

**Mithun** (m) couple, union

**Mitraa** (f) sun **Mitra** (m)

**Mitravindaa** (f) one who gets friends

**Mitravrindaa** (f) a woman who has many friends

**Mitreyu** (m) friendly-minded

**Mitula** (m) limited **Mitulaa** (f)

**Mohaa** (f) embarrassment

**Mohaka** (m) one who is attractive

**Mohana** (m) fascinating

**Mohanaa** (f) one who attracts

**Mohini** (f) one who fascinates

**Mohaangee** (f) one who has an attractive figure

**Mohita** (m) one who is ensnared by beauty

**Monaa** (f) single, alone

**Monal** (f) a bird

**Monisha** (m) lord of mind

**Moraara** (m) peacock

**Motee** (m/f) pearl

**Mrinaalinee/Mrugaakshee/ Mrugalochanaa/Mruga- nayani** (f) doe-eyed

**Mrugaaksha** (m) deer-eye

**Mrudula** (m) tender

**Mrudulaa** (f) delicate woman

**Mrugaa** (f) doe

**Mrugaraaja** (m) king of animals

**Mruda** (m) Shiva

**Mrudaanee** (f) Paarvatee

**Mrugendra** (m) king of animals, the lion

**Mrugesha** (m) lord of animals

**Mrutyunjaya** (m) one who has won victory over death

**Mrunaalee/Mrinali/Mruna- likaa/Mrinaalikaa** (f) lotus stalk

**Mrunaalavatee/Mrinalavatee** (f) like a lotus

**Mukesha** (m) lord of the dumb

**Muktaa** (f) a free soul, pearl

**Muktaavali** (f) a necklace of pearls

**Mukhendu** (m) a moon-like face

**Muktesha** (m) lord of liberated persons

**Mukula** (m) a bud

**Muditaa** (f) one who is pleased

**Mudraa** (f) a seal

**Mudrikaa** (f) a seal, ring
**Mugdhaa** (f) attractive
**Mularaaja** (m) mul    root
**Mulkaraaja** (m) mulk home, village
**Muralee** (m) flute
**Maghavan** (m) Indra

**Maatarishvan**(m) the wind
**Madhavikaa** (f) a creeper
**Murti** (f) source of all qualities
**Moorthy, Moorthi** anything which has a definite shape

# N

Nabhaswatee (f) one who creates sound in the skies

Nabhakaanti (m) splendour of the skies

Nabhamani (m) jewel of the skies, the sun

Nachiketa (m) fire

Naagabhushana (m) one who has a serpent as his ornament

Naagapushpa (f) the champak tree

Naagavalli (f) the naaga creeper. Also Naagalataa

Naagaraaja/Naagendra/ Naagesha (m) king of the serpents

Nagendra (m) lord of the mountains

Nagaja (f) born of the mountain

Naageshwara (m) lord of the cobras

Nakshatra (m) star

Nakshatranaatha/Nakshatrapati (m) lord of the stars, moon

Nakshatramaalaa (f) string of stars

Nalina (m) lotus, water

Nalineei (f) lotus

Naleenaakshee (f) lotus-eyed

Nalinaksha (m)

Nandinee (f) daughter

Namitaa (f) humility

Namrataa (f) humility

Nandana (m) son, pleasing

Nandanaa (f) daughter

Nandi (m) one who pleases others Nanditaa (f)

Navina (m) new, fresh

Neelaanjanaa (f) black surma

Nibhaa (f) light, similar

Nidhisha (m) lord of treasure

Nimeelaa (f) pretence

Ninaada (m) sound, noise

Nipa (m) kadamba tree

Nipaa (f)

Nishita (m) midnight

Niteesha (m) lord of the rule of law

Nivraanshu (m) rays of the moon

Nara (m) literally, man

Narottama (m) best among men

Narasimha (m) lion among men

Naaraayana (m) refuge of man

Naren/Naresha/Narendra (m) king among men

Naaraayanee (f) one who has a house in water

Narahari (m) man-lion

Naaree (f) woman

Narmada (m) bringing delight

Narmadaa (f) a holy river in India

Nata (m) a dancer, an actor

Natee (f)

Nataraaja (m) king among actors

Navakaalikaa (f) a newly-married woman

Nayana (m) eye Nayanaa (f)

**Navamallikaa** (f) a variety of jasmine

**Navanidhiana** (m) one having nine different treasures

**Navanita** (m) fresh butter

**Nayanataaraa** (f) eyes like stars

**Neela** (m) blue **Neelaa** (f)

**Neerajaa** (f) lotus

**Neelam** (f) emerald

**Neelimaa** (f) blue complexioned

**Neelakantha** (m) peacock

**Neeraajanaa** (f) act of adoration

**Netraa** (f) eye

**Netramatee** (f) one with eyes filled with beauty

**Nidhi** (m) the ocean, one endowed with good qualities

**Nidhishwara** (m) lord of the treasure

**Nighna** (m) dependent on

**Nihaara** (m) fog, mist

**Nihaarikaa** (f) heavy dew

**Nijaa** (f) one's own

**Niketa** (m) house, habitation

**Niketana** (m) a mansion

**Nikhila** (m) complete, whole

**Nipunaa** (f) clever, sharp

**Nimilaa/Nimilikaa** (f) shutting the eyes

**Nikulaa/Nikulinikaa** (f) a family art inherited by birth

**Nikunja** (f) a bower

**Neelaakshee** (f) blue-eyed

**Neelaambaree** (f) one dressed in dark blue clothes

**Neelaanga** (m) blue-complexioned

**Neelaanjana** (m) antimony

**Nilaya** (m) heaven

**Nishka** (m) ornament

**Neelendra** (m) king of darkness

**Neelesh** (m) blue god

**Nimi** (m) wink

**Nilimpaa** (f) name of a holy cow

**Niraad** (m) given by water

**Ninaada** (m) gentle murmur of water

**Nipuna** (m) knowledgeable

**Neerajaa** (f) a lotus

**Nireekshaa** (f) searching

**Nirupana** (f) form, sight

**Nirupamaa** (f) incomparable

**Nishkaama** (m) one without desire

**Niraalee** (f) exceptional

**Niraamayee** (f) pure, clean

**Niranjana** (m) simple

**Niranjanaa** (f) unstained

**Nirmala** (m) pure **Nirmalaa** (f)

**Nirmalendu** (m) clear moon

**Nirmalakumara** (m) clean boy

**Nirupaa** (f) shapeless

**Neerava** (m) without sound

**Nirvaana** (m) final liberation

**Nishaa** (f) night

**Nishatha** (m) polished, bright

**Nishchala** (m) steady

**Nishchalaa** (f)

**Nshchinta** (m) free from anxiety

**Nishikaanta/Nishaakaanta** (m) lord of the night, moon

**Neeti** (f) conduct

**Neetaa** (f) well-behaved

**Neeteepa** (m) one who protects law

**Neetisha** (m) one versed in law, rules

**Nityaa** (f) constant, eternal

**Nityaananda** (m) perennially happy

**Niveditaa** (f) teacher
**Nivrutti** (m) separation from the world
**Niyati** (f) destiny, luck
**Nupra** (f) anklets

**Nrupendra/Nripendra** (m) king of kings
**Nutana** (f) novel, new
**Nishaada** (m) seventh note on the Indian musical scale

# O

**Om** (m) a word of solemn invocation, affirmation, benediction and consent

**Omananda** (m) joy of Om

**Oudichya** (m) living or being in the north **Udichi** (f) northern

**Occhav** (m) festive occasion

**Ogaan**(m) wave

**Oja** (m) brightness

**Ojas** (m) bodily strength

**Ojasvini** (f) an elaborate style

**Ojasvitaa** (f) personality

**Omprakaasha** (m) light of Om

**Oshadhi** (f) a medicinal plant or drug

**Oojam** (m) enthusiasm

**Oordhva** (m) towards the sky

**Oorjita** (m) powerful

**Oormi** (f) current, flow, a term in music

# P

**Padmaa** (f) lotus
**Padmaja/Padmabhoota** (m) born of the lotus
**Padmaasanaa** (f) Lakshmee seated on the lotus
**Padmakaanta** (m) beautiful like the lotus
**Padmamaalaa** (f) garland of lotus flowers
**Padmanaabha** (m) one who has a lotus in his navel
**Padmaanjali** (f) one whose hands are full of lotuses
**Padmarekhaa** (f) a small portion of lotus
**Padminn** (m) an elephant
**Padminee** (f)
**Padmakshee** (f) lotus-eyed
**Padmaksha** (m)
**Padmalataa** (f) a lotus creeper
**Padmalochana** (m) lotus-eyed
**Padmalochanaa** (f)
**Padmalochini** (f)
**Padmapriya** (m) beloved of the lotus **Padmapriyaa** (f)
**Padmaparaaga** (m) pollen of the lotus
**Padmaanana** (m) lotus-faced
**Padmapatraa** (f) Lakshmi
**Padmaprasannaa** (f) pleased by the lotus
**Padmaprasanna** (m)
**Padmaraaga** (m) a ruby
**Padmaaraanee** (f) queen of the lotus
**Padmarupaa** (f) one who has lotus-like beauty
**Padmavarnaa** (f) lotus-colored

**Padmasambhavaa** (f) one born out of the lotus
**Padmashobhaa** (f) shining like a lotus
**Padminee** (f) beautiful
**Palaashikasa** (f) petal of a palashi flower
**Pallavee** (f) creeper in full bloom
**Pallavinee** (f) having young shoots or leaves
**Palli** (f) lamp
**Pallikaa** (f) a small village
**Paranjaya** (m) one who conquers others
**Parabrahmana** (m) the supreme spirit
**Panchabaana** (m) the five arrows
**Panchaalikaa** (f) a doll
**Paanduranga** (m) pale white in complexion
**Pankajaa** (f) born in mud
**Pankajaakshee** (f) lotus-eyed
**Pankajanayanee** (f)
**Pankti** (f) a line
**Pankajinee** (f) lotus plant
**Pannaa** (f) emerald
**Pannagesha** (m) king of serpents
**Parjanya** (m) rain
**Paraaga** (m) pollen
**Paramaartha** (m) highest truth
**Paramajeeta** (m) excellent success
**Paramahamsa** (m) the supreme spirit; a spiritual title

**Parameshtni** (m) great god
**Paramasukha** (m) the ultimate happiness
**Parameshwara** (m) supreme god **Parameshwaree** (f)
**Pariketa** (m) against desire
**Paresha** (m) supreme spirit
**Parimala** (f) a fragrant substance **Parimalaa** (f)
**Parimitaa** (f) moderate
**Paarindra** (m) a lion
**Parineetaa** (f) a married woman
**Paritaa** (f) in each direction
**Parivrittaa** (f) revolved, ended
**Parnaa** (f) leaves
**Paarshada** (m) a companion
**Paarthiva** (m) a king
**Paarthava** (m) greatness
**Parvata** (m) mountain
**Paarvatee** (f) daughter of the mountain
**Pashubharata** (m) lord of all creatures
**Pashupatinaatha** (m) lord of all animals
**Paatali** (f) the trumpet flower
**Pathik** (m) traveller
**Pauraalikaa** (f) a raag
**Paavaka** (m) pure, clear
**Pavanee** (f) wind **Pavana** (m)
**Paavand** (m) pure, chaste, **Paavani** (f)
**Paavana** (m) holy, pure
**Paavanee** (f) sacred
**Pavitree** (f) holy
**Pavitraa** (f) chaste, pure
**Paayala** (f) anklet
**Payaswini** (f) a milch-cow
**Pinaakin** (m) pinakk Shiva's bow
**Pinaakapaani** (m) one who holds the bow

**Pingalaaksha** (m) one having brown eyes
**Pitaamaha** (m) the paternal grandfather
**Putaambara** (m) yellow-robed
**Pivara** (m) stout, fat
**Piyushaa** (f) full of nectar
**Piyusha** (m) milk
**Poojaa** (f) act of worship
**Poonam** (f) night of the full moon
**Poornaa** (f) complete, fulness
**Poornachandra** (m) full moon
**Poorbi** (f) ancient
**Poornajita** (m) total victory
**Poornaananda** (m) complete joy
**Poornashree** (f) full of beauty
**Poornaayu** (m) full of life
**Poornendra** (m) powerful Indra
**Poorvaa** (f) the east
**Poorvajaa** (f) one who comes before
**Poorvasha** (m) lord of the east
**Poorti** (f) fulfilment
**Pooshan** (m) one who nourishes
**Poojya** one worthy of being worshipped
**Pulina** (m)shore, a sandy beach
**Pulinabihaaree** (m) one who amuses himself on the shore
**Pundarika/Punnaaga** (m) white lotus
**Pundarikaa** (f) lotus-like
**Pundarikaaksha** (m) lotus-eyed
**Puneeta** (m) pure **Puneetaa** (f)
**Puneevtavatee** (f) one filled with holiness
**Punyakeerti** (m) literally, fame

46

**Punyavaana** (m) virtuous
**Punyavatee** (f)
**Purandaraa** (f) one who destroys the city
**Purnimaa/Poornimaa** (f) night of the full moon
**Purujeeta** (m) victor over the city
**Puraari** (m) enemy of the city
**Puru** (m) city
**Purumitra** (m) friend of the city
**Paritosha** (m) contentment
**Purushottama** (m) best among men
**Pushkalaa** (f) excellent, rich
**Pushkara** (m) a blue lotus
**Pushkaraaksha** (m) lotus-eyed
**Pushpaa** (f) flower
**Pushpadhara** (m) one who holds a flower
**Pushpaja** (m) the juice of flowers
**Pushpajaa** (f) literally, born of a flower
**Pushpalataa** (f) a flowering creeper
**Pushpaka** (m) a flower
**Pushpamanjaree** (f) a flower-bud
**Pushpamayee** (f) one full of flowers
**Pushpamitra** (m) a friend of flowers
**Pushpaanganaa/Pushpaangee** (f) delicate as a flower
**Pushpadanta** (m) one who has teeth like petals
**Pushparaaga** (m) a gem
**Pushpasena** (m) lord of flowers
**Pushpendu** (m) white lotus

**Pushparenu** (f) the pollen of flowers
**Pushpashree** (f) the beauty of flowers
**Pushpavallee** (f) a row of flowers
**Pushpendra** (m) king among flowers
**Pushpesha** (m) lord among flowers
**Pushpeekaa** (f) the last words of a chapter which state the subject treated therein
**Pushti** (f) nourishing
**Parivraajaka** (m) sanyasin
**Parnikaa** (f) small leaf
**Paryaya** (m) order
**Pingesha** (m) one who shines
**Pra** as a prefix to verbs, it means forward, forth, in front, onwards, before, away; with adjectives it means very, excessive, very much, with nouns whether derived from verbs or not, it is used in the following senses; beginning, length, power, origin, excess source, completion, apart, excellence, wish.
**Prabhaa/Prabhaasaa** (f) splendour, beauty
**Prabhaagachandra** (m) part of the moon
**Prabhaanaatha** (m) master of light
**Prabhaanka** (m) a mark of light
**Prabhash** (m) a man of many words
**Prabhaata** (m) dawn
**Prabhaatee** (f)
**Prabhavaa** (f) source, origin

47

**Prabhaava** (m) that which existed before

**Prabhaavali** (f) lustre, light

**Prabhaavi** (m) to pass into the future

**Prabhudatta** (m) given by god

**Prabira/Pravira** (m) hero, brave one

**Prabodha** (m) sound advice

**Prabodhinee** (f) awakening

**Prabodhana** (m) knowledge

**Prabhuti** (f) well-being

**Prakaashati** (f) shines

**Prabuddha** (m) very intelligent

**Praachee** (f) the eastern horizon

**Praacheenaa** (f) ancient

**Pracheetaa** (f) chit pure intelligence, the soul

**Prachetas** (m) chetas sense, mind, reasoning faculty

**Pradeepa** (m) to shine

**Pradhaa** (f) to place, set

**Praduptaa** (f) blazing, illuminated

**Pradyota** (m) exceedingly bright

**Praphulla/Prafulla** (m) pleasant, cheerful

**Praphulla/Prafullaa** (f)

**Praphullavadanaa** (f) one with a pleasant face

**Pragati** (f) progress

**Prajnesha** (m) lord of wisdom

**Prajnaa** (m) insight, wisdom

**Pragnyee** (f) witty, intelligent

**Prajnayaruchi** (f) worship of knowledge

**Pragnyataa** (f) wisdom

**Pragnyakara** (m) one who is very intelligent

**Prahlaada** (m) excess of joy

**Praharshaa** (f) one who is joyous and happy

**Prajeet** (m) victorious

**Prajesha** (m) lord of the people

**Prakaasha** (m) light

**Prakaashaaditya** (m) the bright sun

**Prakaashini** (f) dazzling

**Praalambha** (m) taking hold of

**Pramaadhana** (m) wealth of laziness

**Pramatha** (m) a horse

**Pramathana** (m) Shiva

**Pramathanaatha** (m) king of horses

**Pramesha** (m) master of accurate knowledge

**Pramati** (m) very intelligent

**Pramita** (m) consciousness

**Pramoda** (m) happiness, joy

**Pramodaa** (f)

**Pramodana** (m) gladdening

**Pramodini** (f)

**Praana** (m) life, vital air

**Pranaati** (f) a bow, courtesy

**Praananaatha** (m) lord of life

**Pranava** (m) the sacred syllable Om

**Pranavaa** (f) young

**Pranavaanjali** (f) respectful salutation

**Pranayinke** (f) beloved

**Praneta** (m) leader

**Pranetaa** (f)

**Pratimaa** (f) an image, statue

**Praarthanaa** (f) prayer

**Praanjala** (f) honest, sincere

**Praanjali** (f) an act of joining two hands together

**Pranoti/Pranati** (f) humility

**Praapti** (f) attainment

**Prasaada** (m) offering
**Prasanna** (m) pleased
**Prashaanta** (m) very calm and composed **Prashaanti** (f)
**Prashamsaa** (f) praise, glory
**Pragalbhaa** (f) brave, bold
**Prasooti** (f) sooti    to give birth
**Prataapa** (m) dignity, majesty
**Prateechi** (f) western direction
**Prateeka** (m) first word in a sentence
**Pratima** (m) comparable
**Praphullataa** (f) a creeper full of flowers
**Prasoona** (m) flower
**Preeyaati** (f) dearly beloved
**Prathamesha** (m) most excellent master
**Prathithi** (f) famous
**Prathithaa** (f) renowned
**Pratibhaa** (f) light, genius
**Pratikaami** (m) desirous
**Pratikshaa** (f) hope
**Pratirupaa** (f) resemblance of beauty
**Pratosha** (m) extreme delight
**Pratulachandra** (m) incomparable moon
**Prathushti** (f) extreme satisfaction
**Pratyusha** (m) the rising sun
**Pravaraa** (f) chief, principal
**Pravassee** (f) traveller
**Pravaasinee** (f)
**Praveni** (f) a braid of hair
**Pravinaa** (m) clever
**Pravina** (m) expert
**Priyaanka** (m) very dear husband
**Pravara** (m) chief
**Pravinasaagara** (m) pravin skilled, saagar    sea

**Pravira** (m) brave
**Prayaati** (f) advanced, dead
**Preetaatmaa** (m) one with a loving heart
**Preeti** (f) love, happiness
**Preetitosha** (m) pleasure of love
**Preetivardana** (m) one who increases love
**Prekshaa** (f) wise
**Prema** (m) love **Premaa** (f)
**Premajaa** (f) born of love
**Premala** (m) full of love
**Premaananda** (m) joy of love
**Premasaagara** (m) sea of love
**Premendra** (m) king of love
**Premanivaasa** (f) house of love
**Premvalli** (f) creeper of love
**Preranaa** (f) encouragement
**Preyaa** (f) more beloved
**Preyasa** (m) one who tries to get material enjoyment for himself
**Pritam** (m) lover
**Prithviraja** (m) king of the world
**Prithu** (m) broad, spacious
**Pruthulomaa** (f) one having long hair
**Pruthushekhara** (m) mountain having wide summit
**Pruthushree** (f) highly prosperous
**Prithveevallabha** (m) master of the world
**Pritisha** (m) lord of love
**Priyaa** (f) lover
**Priyadarshana** (m) good-looking
**Priyadarshanaa/Priyadarshinee** (f) beautiful
**Priyam** (m) dear, beloved

**Priyammayaa/Priyaamaya (f)**
full of love

**Priyamvadaa (f)** soft spoken

**Priyankaa (f)** one with a
beautiful mark

**Priyanakara (m)** lover

**Priyankaree (f)**

**Prithvi (f)** the earth

**Priyaamshu (m)** one wearing
a beautiful garment

**Priyaranjana (m)** beloved

**Priyataa (f)** being dear

**Priyavadana (m)** one having
a lovely face

**Pruthvisha (m)** lord of the
earth

# R

Rachanaa (f) arrangement
Paadhaa (f) prosperity
Raadhikaa (f) Raadhaa
Raaga (f) a musical note
Raaja (m) king
Raanee (f) queen
Rajanee (f) night
Rajaneekaanta (m) lord of the
  night
Raajakumaara (m) prince
Raajaamsaa (m) a flamingo
Raajanvatee (f) the earth,
  governed by a good king
Raajakumari/Raajadulaaree
  (f) a princess
Raajyavardhana (m) one who
  increases the prosperity of a
  kingdom
Raajavilochana (m) one
  having beautiful eyes
Raajyashree (f) prosperity of
  a king
Raajyavatee (f) one who owns
  a kingdom
Raakesha (m) lord of the
  night
Raakhaala (m) derived from
  raksha    to save, protect
Ramaa (f) beautiful
Ramanakaantaa (f) charming
Ramana (m) beloved, pleasing
Ramanaa/Ramanee (f)
  beautiful
Ramanika (m) handsome
Ramanikaa (f)
Ramanimohana (m) one who
  charms a beautiful woman
Raajeeva (m) a blue lotus

Rajeevalochan (m) lotus-eyed
Ramita (m) omnipresent
Ramitaa (f)
Ramonaa (f) protector
Ramyaa (f) pleasing woman
Ravindra (m) the sun lord
Rashanaa (m) woman's girdle
Raamakumaar (m) kumaara
  boy, youth
Raamamohana (m) literally,
  delight of Raama
Raamaprasaada (m) blessings
  of Raama
Ramachhoda (m) one who
  leaves the field
Ramaveera (m) hero of the
  battle
Rangabihaaree (m) one who
  plays with colours
Ranganaa (f) ranga    colour
Rangati (f) a classical melody
Ranjana (m) pleasing, delight-
  ing Ranjanaa (f)
Ranjeekaa (f) one of the
  shrutis
Ranjitaa (f) to fall in love
  with
Ranajeeta (m) victorious on
  the battlefield
Rathin (m) warrior
Rathindra (m) king of
  warriors
Rujutaa (f) sincerity
Rujusmitaa (f) one having a
  sober smile
Rujusmriti (f) one having
  sober memory
Ratnamani (m) precious stone

**Rasajnaa** (f) knowledgeable about different arts

**Rasesha** (m) lord of taste (rasa-taste)

**Rashmi** (m/f) ray of the early morning sun

**Rashmimohana** (m) one who delights in the early morning's sun's ray

**Rashmikaa** (f) a tiny ray of light

**Rashmikaanta** (m) lord of the ray

**Rashmikety** (m) one who has a banner of rays

**Rasika** (m) one who appreciates excellence or beauty

**Ratnam** a precious stone, a jewel

**Ratiramana** (m) god of love

**Ratnaakaras** (m) mine of jewels

**Ratnamaalaa** (f) a string of precious stones

**Ratnaprabhaa** (f) lustre of jewels

**Ratnapriyaa** (f) beloved of the gems

**Ratnasambhava** (m) one born of precious stones

**Ratnaavalee** (f) necklace of jewels

**Raatri** (f) night

**Ratnaangee** (f) jewelled limbs

**Ravi** (m) a particular aspect of the sun

**Ravibaalaa** (f) daughter of the sun

**Ravija** (m) born of the sun

**Ravijaa** (f)

**Ravikirana** (m) ray of the sun

**Ravinaatha** (m) lotus

**Ravikeerti** (m) one whose fame is like the sun

**Raviranjana** (m) dazzling as the sun

**Ravisha** (m) lord of the sun

**Raviraaja** (m) sun king

**Renu** (m/f) dust, atom

**Rekhaa** (f) a line, a streak

**Revatee** (f) prosperity

**Riddi** (f) prosperity, success

**Rishab** (m) morality

**Rishabhadaeva** (m) lord of morality

**Rishikulyaa** (f)   virtuous

**Rishiraaja** (m) king among ascetics

**Rochanaa** (f) splendid, beautiful

**Rochana** (m) red lotus, bright

**Rochanee** (f) beautiful

**Ritikaa** (f) moving, flowing

**Rochiraa** (f) light, glow

**Rochisha** (m) light, brightness

**Rochishaa** (f)

**Rohita** (m) red

**Rokshadaa** (f) possessing light

**Romaa** (f) a hairy woman

**Romaharsha** (f) bristling of the hair in delight

**Roopa** (f) shape, one who is beautiful

**Roopakoshaa** (f) treasure of beauty

**Roopalekhaa** (f) streak of beauty

**Rooparashmi** (f) rays of beauty

**Ruchaa** (f) light, lustre

**Ruchira** (m) handsome, shining **Ruchiraa** (f)

**Ruchi/Ruchikaa/Ruchilaa** (f) beautiful, attractive

**Rukma** (m) gold
**Rupam** (m) beauty, form
**Rupamanjaree** (f) sprout of beauty
**Rupaambaraa/Rupaambaree** (f) one dressed in beautiful clothes
**Rupaka** (m) a sign, feature
**Rupala** (f) made of silver
**Rupaalee** (f) beautiful girl
**Rupanga** (m) silver-bodied
**Rupaangee/Rupaanginee** (f)
**Rupaavatee** (f) full of beauty
**Rupesha** (m) lord of beauty
**Rupeshwaree** (f) goddess of beauty
**Rupalataa** (f) creeper of beauty
**Rupalatikaa** (f) a small creeper of beauty
**Rupalekhaa** (f) a streak of beauty
**Rupashree** (f) beautiful Lakshmi
**Rupin** (m) embodied beauty
**Rujula** (m) uncomplicated
**Rujulaa** (f) simple, honest
**Ruksharaa** (f) flow of water

**Rukshesha** (m) king of stars, moon
**Rushi** (m) a sage, ray of light
**Rushikaanta** (m) lord of the ascetics
**Ruchika** (m) a sage
**Ruddhidaa** (f) one who endows prosperity
**Ruju** (m) plain or simple
**Rujaraaja** (m) moon
**Rushiraaja** (m) king of the ascetics
**Rutaa** (f) also Rtaa, honest woman
**Rushyashringa** (m) deer-horned
**Rutajaa** (f) daughter of truth
**Rutajeet** (m) conqueror of truth
**Rutujeet** (m) one who conquers the six seasons
**Rutumbharaa** (f) one who bears divine truth
**Rutunjaya** (m) one who conquers the seasons
**Rutushree** (f) splendour of the seasons
**Rutvija** (m) a priest who officiates at a sacrifice

# S

Sachchidaananda (m) joy of the supreme spirit

Sachi (m) a friend

Sadaananda (m) ever joyous

Saadhanaa (f) fulfilment

Saadhikaa (f) a skilful or accomplished woman

Saadhuraama (m) noble, virtuous

Saagara (m) ocean

Saguna (m) virtuous

Sagunaa (f)

Sahajaananda (m) natural joy

Sahasrabaahu (m) a thousand-armed

Sahasrajita (m) one who has conquered thousands of enemies

Sahasraamshu (m) the sun

Sahishnu (m/f) capable of enduring

Sahasraaksha (m) thousand-eyed

Shailesha (m) the Himalaya

Saimyama (m) restraint

Samyuktaa (f) joined

Sajanee (f) virtuous

Sajjana (m)

Saakara (m) sugar

Sakulaa (f) belonging to a noble family

Salila (m) water

Salonee (f) beautiful

Salonavaira (m) handsome

Samaa (m) equal, same

Samitaa (f) wheat flour

Samaapati (f) the end

Samichi (m) going with; right

Sama as a prefix to verbs and verbal derivatives to mean: with, together with, and as prefix to nouns to mean: like, same, similar

Sambhooti (f) knowledge; birth, origin; union

Saakambharee (f) herb-bearing

Samiraa (f) wind Samira (m)

Sammardana (m) rubbing together

Sampurnaananda (m) fullest joy

Sampuranaa (f) total, complete

Samudraa (f) ocean

Samyaati (f) to accompany

Sanaatana (m) constant, firm

Sanchitaa (f) one who collects

Sandeepa (m) a lighted lamp

Sandeepana/Sandipani (m) kindling, inflaming

Sandhyaa (f) twilight

Sanghabhuti (m) collection of wealth

Sangharakhshita (m) protected by a group

Sangati (m) union, company

Sangatikaa (f) term used in music

Sanginee (f) companion

Sangeeitaa (f) one who knows to sing; music

Sangeeti (f) harmony

Sangraama (m) battle

Sankataharanaa (f) a goddess who destroys all difficulties and obstacles

**Sankalpa** (m) will, volition; intention, purpose

**Sanmitra** (m) a very good friend

**Sanmukha** (m/f) in the presence of; happy visage

**Sannidhi** (m) proximity

**Santosha** (m/f) satisfaction

**Sapana** (m) dream **Sapanaa** (f) (Swapna in Sanskrit)

**Saralaa** (f) simple, honest

**Saarana** (m) causing to go or flow

**Saaranga** (m) the spotted deer

**Saarangpaani** (m) one who holds a deer

**Shaarangapaani** (m) one who holds a bow

**Saarasaa** (m) belonging to a lake (the swan) **Saarasee** (f)

**Samiti** (f) meeting, union

**Samriddhi** (f) prosperity

**Sanidha** (f) firewood

**Samarpanaa** (f) handing over, dedicating

**Samaa** (m) a year

**Saaraswata** (m) learned

**Saraswatee** (f) watery; elegant

**Sarayu** (f) air, wind

**Saarikaa** (f) a bird

**Saritaa** (f) to flow; a river

**Saroja** (f) lotus

**Sarojinee** (f) cluster of lotuses

**Sarva** (m) whole, entire

**Sarvadamana** (m) literally, one who subdues everyone

**Sarvajnya** (m) omniscient

**Sarvamangalaa** (f) one who brings good fortune to all

**Sarvananadin** (m) one who pleases all

**Sarvaavasu** (m) wealth, riches

**Satee** (f) chaste, austere

**Sarvayasha** (m) the whole fame

**Sarvottama** (m) best among all

**Satdhruti** (m) a truly bold person

**Shabalaa/Shabali** (f) a spotted or brindled cow

**Shaachee/Shachee** (f) speech, eloquence

**Shadabhujaa** (f) a goddess having six arms

**Shadri** (f) a cloud; lightning; an elephant

**Sadaanana** (m) one having six faces

**Shafar** (m) fish **Shafaree** (f)

**Shaadhwal** (m) with green grass

**Shag** (m) flame of a lamp

**Shaila** (m) mountain

**Shailaa** (f)

**Shailabaalaa** (f) daughter of the mountain

**Shailajaa** (f) born of the mountain

**Shailaka** (m) benzoin; bitumen

**Shailaalin** (m) actor, dancer

**Shailaalika** (m) range of mountains

**Shailen/Shailendra** (m) king of mountains. Himalaya

**Shailesha** (m) king of mountain **Shaileshee** (f)

**Shaileya** (m) full of mountains

**Shailee** (f) a mode of expression or interpretation; behaviour, conduct

**Shaishava** (m) childhood

**Shaitya** (m) cold; frigidity

**Shakan/Shakun** (m/f) good omen

**Shakaari** (m) enemy of the Shaka tribe

**Shakata** (m) cart

**Shakra** (m) an owl; the number '14'

**Sakree** (m) an elephant; a mountain; a cloud

**Shakti** (f) power; ability

**Shaktikumaara** (m) powerful and young

**Shakraaditya** (m) radiant as the sun

**Shakuni** (f) a bird

**Shakunikaa** (f) a sparrow

**Shakunta/Shakuntak** (m) good omen; the blue jay

**Shakunti** (f) bird

**Shakuntikaa** (f) a bird

**Shala** (m) a dart, spear

**Shaalabhanjikaa** (f) a doll

**Shalaakaa** (f) small, thin stick

**Shashikaant** (m) the moon gem

**Shaaligraama** (m) a black, smooth, rounded stone

**Shaalihotree** (m) veterinarian

**Shaalikaa** (f) parrot, weaver

**Shaalin** (m/f) modest, noble

**Shaalinaa** (f) domestic

**Shaalinee** (f) housewife

**Shaalmala** (m) the cotton tree

**Shaalmali** (m) the silk cotton tree

**Shalya** (m) a shaft, an arrow

**Shalyaa** (f) a slab of stone

**Shalyaka** (m) a dart; javelin

**Shama** (m) tranquillity; peace

**Shamaa** (f) flame; candle

**Shaamaa/Shyamaa** (f) night; shade; shadow

**Shamataa** (f) peace; patience; forgiveness. **Shaman** (m)

**Shambari** (f) illusion, jugglery

**Shambhu** (m) the iron head of a pestle

**Shambhuprasaada** (m) gift of a happy man

**Shaamaka** (m) calming, pacifying

**Shaminn** (m) calm, peaceful

**Shamita** (m) calmed

**Shamitaa** (f)

**Shammarda** (m) joyous

**Shamsukha** (m) peace of mind

**Shanavi** (m) one who can read and tell about auspicious moments and days

**Shaangar** (m) bow of Vishnu

**Shani** (m) the planet Saturn

**Shankara** (m) auspicious; giver of joy and happiness

**Shankha** (m) a shell

**Shankhalee** (m) a small shell

**Shanku** (m) a dart, spear

**Shaantaa** (f) peaceful

**Shaantataa** (f) peace

**Shaanti** (f) peace, quiet

**Shaantidaa** (f) one who gives peace

**Shantideva** (m) god of peace

**Shaantidevi** (f)

**Shaantiprasaada** (m) blessing of calmness

**Shara** (m) an arrow

**Sharabhaa** (f) young elephant

**Sharabhu** (m) one born of an arrow

**Sharada** (m/f) one of the six seasons

**Shaaradaa** (f) goddess of knowledge

**Sharandi** (m) a quiver

**Sharadamani** (f) mani    jewel

**Sharana** (m) shelter, refuge

**Shaardula** (m) a tiger; an eminent person

**Sharanee** (f) earth; a pathway

**Sharata** (m) a challenge

**Sharanya** (m) one who can protect

**Sharma** (m) joy, happiness

**Sharmada** (m) giver of peace and joy **Sharmadaa** (f)

**Sharaprabhaava** (m) power of the arrow

**Sharvila** (m) Shiva

**Sharvari** (f) night

**Sharvareesha** (m) lord of the night; moon

**Shashee** (m) moon

**Shashaanka** (m) the moon

**Shashibindu** (m) bindu spot

**Shashilekhaa** (m) a digit of the moon; moonlight

**Shashikaanta** (m) the moon-stone **Shashikaantaa** (f)

**Shashikara** (m) moon

**Shashimi** (f) hare

**Shashimukhee** (f) moon-faced

**Shashin** (m) hare-marked; the moon **Shashinee** (f)

**Shashiprabhaa** (f) light of the moon

**Shashisha** (m) Lord of the moon

**Shaastaa** (m) king, teacher

**Shaashwata** (m) continuous

**Shasshwatee** (f) eternal

**Shaataa** (f) peace

**Shatabindu** (m) a shower of raindrops

**Shatadanva** (m) one who has hundreds of bows

**Shatajeeta** (m) one who conquers hundreds

**Shatajyoti** (f) bright as hundred flames

**Shatakratu** (m) one who performs a hundred sacrifices

**Shataakshee** (f) one who has a hundred eyes

**Shataanan** (m) one who has a hundred faces

**Shataananyda** (m) extremely joyful

**Shatanika** (m) an old man

**Shatvaree** (f) night

**Shatisha/Satish** (m) ruler of hundreds

**Shatrajeet** (m) victor over hundreds

**Shatrunjaya** (m) one who overcomes enemies

**Shatrupaala** (m) one who protects his enemy

**Shaavaka** (m) child

**Shayyaa** (f) a bed, companionship

**Sheelabhadra** (m) one having good character

**Sheelavanti** (f) a good character

**Sheetaabha** (m) cold lustre

**Sheetabindu** (m) cold drop

**Sheetala** (f) cool

**Shefaali** (f) a kind of plant

**Shefaalika** (f)

**Sheila** (m) mountain

**Sheilaa** (f)

**Shikhaa** f) small plait of hair; top, summit

**Shilaali** (m) line of stones

**Sheelaa** (m) one who has good character

**Sheshaadri** (m) shesha    rest; adri    mountain

**Shekhara** (m) a diadem or ornament representing the crescent of the fifth day moon

**Shilpaa** (f) one who is skilled in any art

**Shishira** (m) cold, frigid

**Shilavantee** (m) possessing moral precepts

**Shishuka** (m) a child

**Shitradri** (m) the cold mountains

**Shitina** (m) one who sharpens his weapons

**Shiva** (m) auspicious; lucky

**Shivaa** (f) Paarvati

**Shivaanee** (f) Paarvatee

**Shivaprasaada** (m) blessings of Shiva

**Shivashree** (m) glory of Shiva

**Shlishaa** (f) embrace

**Shobhaa** (f) light, beauty

**Shobhana** (m) splendid, handsome

**Shobhanee** (f) beautiful

**Shobhanaa** (f) to shine

**Shobhinee** (f) beautiful

**Shobhita** (m) decorated

**Shobhitaa/Sobitaa/Sabita** (f)

**Shonaa** (f) red, crimson

**Shraddhaa** (f) faith; devotion

**Shraddhaananda** (m) delight in faith

**Shravana** (m) lunar mansion containing three stars

**Shraavanee** (f) the day of full moon in the month of Shraavana

**Shree/Shri** (f) prosperity

**Shreebaanee** (f) beautiful language

**Shreebhu** (f) beautiful place

**Shreedaam** (m) beautiful garland

**Shreedarshan** (m) beautiful vision

**Shreedevee** (f) goddess of wealth

**Shreelaa** (f) rich, famous

**Shreedhara** (m) one who holds wealth **Shreedharaa** (f)

**Shridautamaan** (m) purified wealth

**Shreekunja** (f) beautiful place overgrown with plants

**Shreelataa** (f) beautiful, celebrated

**Shreelaabha** (m) acquisition of wealth

**Shreemaana** (m) a wealthy person

**Shreemani** (f) jewel

**Shreematee** (f) wealthy

**Shreeneelaa** (f) a dark-blue beauty

**Shreenidhi** (m) treasure house of wealth

**Shreepaala** (m) one who protects wealth

**Shreepushpa** (m) cloves

**Shreeparnaa** (f) lotus

**Shreeranjanaa** (f) one who gives pleasure

**Shreeranjana** (m)

**Shreesha** (m) lord of wealth

**Shreeshaa** (f)

**Shreevardhana** (m) one who increases wealth

**Shrenee** (f) a line, row

**Shrenika** (m) a flock, group

**Shreya** (m) better

**Shreyaa** (f)

**Shreyas** (m) superior

**Shrungari** (f) decorated

**Shruta** (m) reported, heard

**Shrutaa** (f)

**Shrutaavatee** (f) proficient in the sacred knowledge

**Shruti** (f) having a knowledge of the Vedas

**Shrutakeerti** (f) famous

**Shubhaa** (f) lustre; beauty

**Shubhadaa** (f) one who gives happiness

**Shubhaanga** (m) handsome

**Shuchi** (m) pure, bright

**Shucheendra** (m) lord of purity **Shucheendraa** (f)

**Shubhraa** (f) crystal

**Shuchitaa** (f) purity

**Shuddhaa** (f) pure, clean

**Shuddhimaan** (m) very pure

**Shuka** (m) a parrot

**Shuklaa** (f) white

**Shurottama** (m) best among the brave

**Shwetaa** (f) a cowrie

**Shwetala** (f) white

**Shwetaanga** (m) fair-complexioned **Shwetaange** (f)

**Shwetalataa** (f) a white creeper

**Shwitaan** (m) white

**Shwiti** (f) whiteness

**Shyaama** (m) black; dark blue

**Shyaamaa** (f) night, shadow

**Shyaamala** (m) dark blue

**Shyaamalaa** (f)

**Shyaamalaangee** (f) a dark-complexioned body

**Shyaamalataa** (f) dark colored creeper

**Shyamarupaa** (f) a black beauty

**Siddhaartha** (m) white mustard

**Sindhu** (f) the sea; ocean

**Sindhujaa** (f) born of the ocean

**Siddhi** (f) completion; perfection

**Siddhidaa** (f) one who bestows success

**Siddhikaa** (f) small fulfillment

**Sinduraa** (f) name of a tree

**Shansaa** (f) praise, wish

**Shatrunjaya** (m) victory over the enemy

**Shasyamanjari** (f) an ear of corn

**Shaardula** (m) tiger

**Shaaradi** (f) the full moon day in the month of Kaartik

**Shaashvati** (f) the earth

**Seeta** (f) a furrow personified as a goddess and worshipped as the deity presiding over agriculture

**Sitaamshu** (m) one having white rays; the moon

**Skanda** (m) leaping

**Smitaa** (f) smiling

**Smruti/Smriti** (f) remembrance

**Snehaa** (f) affectionate; oily

**Snehajaa** (f) born from love

**Snehala** (m/f) affectionate

**Snehalataa** (f) creeper of friendship

**Snehaanjali** (f) cavity full of love

**Snehaankitaa** (f) won by love

**Snehann** (m) love, affection

**Somsahree** (f) moon beauty

**Sonaa** (f) gold

**Sonala** (f) of gold: golden

**Sukanyaa** (f) beautiful maiden

**Sujeeta** (m) victory

**Sujaataa** (f) one of high birth

**Sujanaa** (f) good, virtuous

**Suhaasa** (m) one with a lovely winsome smile

**Suhaasinee** (f)

**Subhasini** (f) one who speaks sweetly

**Suhaataa** (f) beautiful

**Sukeshinee** (f) one with lovely hair

**Sugreeva** (m) having a graceful and shapely neck

**Sashitala** (m) very cool
**Subaahu** (m) strong-armed
**Subala** (m) very powerful
**Subhaga** (m) blessed
**Subhagaa** (f) one well-loved by her husband; blessed
**Subhadraa** (f) very prosperous
**Subhaagee** (f) born to good fortune
**Subhaasha** (m) soft-spoken
**Subandhu** (m) having a good connection of friends
**Subhru** (f) one with fine eyebrows
**Subhuti** (f) one enjoying prosperity
**Subhira/Subira/Suvira** (m) good and courageous
**Subodha** (m) easily understood; sound advice
**Subodhinee** (f) clever; shrewd
**Sucharitaa** (f) well-behaved
**Suchetaa** (f) one with a very fine mind
**Suchira** (m) eternity
**Suchiraa** (f)
**Suchita** (m) one who has a noble mind **Suchitaa** (f)
**Sudarshana** (m) good-looking
**Sudhaa** (f) nectar; well-being
**Sudhaakara** (m) a mine of nectar
**Sudaamaa** (m) meek
**Shuddhasattwa/Shuddasattwa** (m) one having a pure existence
**Sudeepta** (m) shining, beautiful **Sudeepti** (f)
**Sudeshakumaara** (m) son of a good country
**Sudhanvaa** (m) an excellent archer
**Sudhaamshu** (m) the moon

**Sudheesha** (m) lord of excellent intellect
**Sudheera** (m) resolute; brave
**Sudhyumna** (m) very bright
**Sugandhaa** (f) sweet smelling
**Sugati** (m) in a good or happy condition
**Sukeshaa** (f) having beautiful hair **Sukesha** (m)
**Sulabhaa** (f) easily obtainable
**Sulabha** (m)
**Sulakshanaa** (f) having an auspicious mark
**Suketu** (m) one having a beautiful flag or banner
**Sukhadeva** (m) god of happiness
**Sukhadevaprasaada** (m) gift of the god of happiness
**Sukeerti** (f) famous
**Sukriti** (m) holy and pure
**Sukshamaa** (f) minute, subtle
**Sukumaara** (m) handsome
**Sulalita** (m) sporting gracefully
**Sulalitaa** (f) dainty
**Sulataa** (f) beautiful creeper
**Sulekhaa** (f) beautiful line
**Sulochana** (m) having beautiful eyes **Sulochanaa** (f)
**Sumaali** (m) well garlanded
**Sumana** (m/f) a flower
**Sumangala** (m) very auspicious **Sumangalaa** (f)
**Sumantra** (m) a good adviser
**Sumantu** (m) a good adviser
**Sumati** (f) with a good mind
**Sumedhaa** (f) sensible
**Sumeghaa** (f) beautiful cloud
**Sumesha** (m) king of flowers
**Sumitaa** (f) well-measured
**Sumitra** (m) good friend
**Sumitraa** (f)

**Sumukhee** (f) beautiful-faced
**Sumukhi** (m)
**Sunanda** (m) one who delights
**Sunandaa** (f)
**Sunandana** (m) delightful son
**Sunandinee** (f)
**Sunandita** (m) one who is joyful **Sunanditaa** (f)
**Sundara** (m) attractive
**Sundaree** (f)
**Sunetraa** (f) having beautiful eyes
**Suneela** (m) dark-blue
**Suneelaa** (f)
**Sunita** (m) well-behaved
**Sunitaa** (f)
**Sunitee** (f) good conduct
**Suparna** (m) having good or beautiful wings
**Suprabhaataa** (f) beautiful dawn
**Suprateem** (m) excellent
**Supreeta** (m/f) well-loved
**Supriya** (m) much loved
**Supriyaa** (f)
**Supushpa** (m) beautiful flower
**Sura** (m) the sun; a hero; wise or learned man
**Surabhi** (f) sweet-smelling
**Surabhitaa** (f) scented
**Suraja** (m/f) the sun
**Surllpriyaa** (f) loved by the gods
**Suraari** (m) enemy of the gods
**Surasaa** (f) juicy; well-flavoured
**Surati** (f) rich in gifts
**Surekha** (m) beautiful
**Surekhaa** (f)
**Surupaa** (f) beautiful
**Surya** (m) the sun
**Suryaa** (f)
**Suryamukhee** (f) sunflower

**Suryabhaa** (f) bright as the sun
**Sughoshaa** (f) pleasant and auspicious sound
**Sughosha** (m)
**Suryakaanta** (m) loved by the sun **Suryakaantaa** (f)
**Suryamohana** (m) beautiful sun
**Suseemaa** (f) cold, pleasant
**Sushamaa/Sushmaa** (f) exquisite beauty
**Sushaanta** (m) appeased
**Susheela** (m) of good disposition **Susheelaa** (f)
**Sushiraa** (f) full of holes
**Sushruta** (m) having a good reputation
**Sushree** (f) excellent beauty
**Susmitaa** (f) one with a smiling countenance
**Suvapu** (f) one who has a beautiful figure
**Suvarnaa** (f) golden complexioned **Suvarna** (m)
**Suvaasinee** (f) one residing in her father's house; a term of courtesy for a married woman whose husband is alive
**Suveera/Suvir/Subir** (m) having brave offspring
**Suvrata/Subrata** (m) strict in observing religious vows
**Suvrataa** (f) a virtuous wife
**Suyama** (m) well-restrained
**Suyashaa** (f) very famous
**Suyodhana** (m) an excellent warrior
**Svaati** (f) a sword
**Swaaminee** (f) an owner
**Swaahaa** (f) an offering made to all gods

**Swapna** (m) dream
**Swapnaa** (f)
**Swapnasundaree** (f) the dream beauty
**Swapneela** (m) seen in a dream
**Swaarbhaanu** (m) the heavenly sun
**Swarnaa** (f) a golden beauty
**Swaroopa** (f) beauty
**Swarooparanee** (f) queen of beauty
**Swarupaa** (f) beautiful
**Swastikaa** (f) a lucky object
**Swayambhu** (m) self-existent
**Swayamjyoti** (f) self-luminous
**Shwetambara** (m) white-clad
**Samvardhana** (m) to grow
**Satkruti** (m) hospitality
**Satvamatee** (f) one endowed with riches
**Satva** (m) spirit; vitality
**Satya** (m) true, genuine
**Satyaa** (f) truthfulness
**Satyakaama** (m) lover of truth
**Satyadaa** (f) one who gives truth
**Satyadeepa** (m) lamp of truth
**Satyadeva** (m) god of truth
**Satyajita** (m) victory of truth
**Satyadhriti** (m) delight of truth
**Satyamurti** (m) statue of truth
**Satyaprema** (m) love of truth
**Satyapriya** (m) one who loves truth **Satyapriyaa** (f)
**Satyaarka** (m) truth as bright as the sun
**Satyarupaa** (f) truth in the form of woman
**Satyashravaa** (m) truthful
**Satyaswaroopa** (m) form of truth
**Satyaayu** (m) truthful life

**Satyatapaa** (m) one who does penance for truth
**Satyavijaya** (m) one who has won the truth
**Satyavrata** (m) one who has taken the vow of truth
**Satyendra** (m) lord of truth
**Saubhaagyasundari** (f) beauty endowed with good fortune
**Sauhaarda** (m) hearty friendship
**Saumyaa** (f) serene
**Saundaraa** (f) beauty
**Saumyendra** (f) most serene
**Saurava** (m) divine; celestial
**Saurabha** (m) fragrance
**Saurabhee** (f) fragrance
**Savarnaa** (f) one belonging to the same caste
**Savitra** (m) the sun
**Saavitreei** (f) a ray of light
**Savyasaachi** (m) one who can shoot an arrow either by the left or right hand
**Seemaa** (f) limit, boundary
**Senaananda** (m) joy of the army
**Senaa** (m) army
**Sevaalee** (f) green moss
**Sevantee** (f) name of a flower
**Sneha** (f) friendship; love
**Snehapriyaa** (f) dear beloved
**Snehprabhaa** (f) lustre of love
**Snigdhaa** (f) loving
**Snushaa** (f) daughter-in-law
**Sohaagee/Subhaagee** (f) fortunate
**Sohana** (m) good looking
**Sohanaa** (f)
**Sohinee** (f) pretty
**Somaamshu** (m) moonbeam
**Sonaalee/Sonaalikaa/Sonitaa** (f) of gold

**Sthaanu** (m) firm, steady
**Sthiramati** (f) one with a firm mind
**Sthulakesha** (m) one who has plenty of hair
**Strotasvinee** (f) flow of water
**Stuti** (f) a song, an invocation
**Syaala** (m) brother-in-law
**Samapada/Sampati** (m) wealth
**Sampaa** (f) lightning
**Sampurna** (m) whole, entire
**Sampurnaa** (f)
**Sampreeti** (f) acquisition
**Sambhaavanaa** (f) fancy, doubt
**Sammohanaa** (f) fascinating
**Samataa** (f) similarity
**Samayaa** (f) in due time
**Samaraa** (m) war, battle
**Sangeeta** (f) one who sings and knows music very well
**Sachetana** (m) rational
**Sachetanaa** (f) sentiment
**Sanchaari** (m) one who roams
**Sanchaarini** (f)
**Saadhanaa** (f) accomplishment
**Saarikaa** (f) a kind of bird
**Sankalanaa** (f) the act of heaping together
**Sankirtanas** (m) glorification
**Sankirtanaa** (f)
**Sanketa** (m) a sign, gesture
**Sangaanikaa** (f) an excellent, incomparable discourse
**Sakaama** (m) with love
**Sakha** (m) friend
**Sakhi** (f)
**Saguna** (m) possessed of virtuous qualities
**Sagunaa** (f)
**Sanstuti** (f) praise, eulogy
**Samsmriti** (f) remembrance
**Santvanaa** (f) conciliation
**Samvidaa** (f) an agreement

**Saptarshi** (m) seven sages; the seven stars in heaven
**Samvidhaa** (f) preparation
**Samvedanaa** (f) knowledge
**Samyogitaa** (f) united
**Sanaapini** (f) speaker
**Samyata** (m) restrained
**Samyamita** (m) bound
**Sarvadaa** (f) always
**Sarveshwara** (m) lord of all
**Sarveshwaree** (f)
**Sushobhana** (m) very handsome **Sushobhanaa** (f)
**Sarasi** (f) a lake, pool
**Sarasija** (f) born in a pool
**Sarasijaaksha** (f) lotus-eyed
**Saritaa** (f) a river
**Sarvasahaa** (f) the earth, one who bears all
**Shankulaa** (f) a pair of scissors
**Shaakunta** (m) the blue jay
**Shakuna** (m) a kind of bird
**Saphala** (m) fruitful
**Saphalaa** (f)
**Shikshaa** (f) discipline; teaching
**Shikarini** (f) pointed
**Shilpaa** (f) one who is an expert in the fine arts
**Shinjini** (f) a bow-string; an anklet
**Shinjaa** (f) tinkle, jingle
**Shlaaghaa** (f) praise
**Shvetaanka** (m) one having a white mark
**Shreemati** (f) wealthy
**Shubhendu** (m) beautiful moon
**Samarjit** (m) victorious in war
**Shubaanana** (m) one who has a handsome face
**Shubaananda** (m) pure joy

**Shushiraa** (f) a river
**Shraddhaa** (f) trust, faith
**Shruti** (f) report, the veda
**Snehini** (f) a friend
**Spanditaa** (f) throbbed, quivered
**Spardhaa** (f) rivalry, competition
**Spardhini** (f) emulating
**Snigdhaa** (f) loving, friendly
**Snehaa** (f) affection, love
**Snehalaa** (f) loving
**Spruhaa** (f) desire
**Sphruti** (f) looming, shaking
**Sevaa** (f) service
**Sthiraa** (f) firm, the earth
**Swaraj** (m) liberty, freedom
**Stimita** (m) still, calm
**Stuti** (f) praise, eulogy

**Simantini** (f) a married woman
**Sitaamshu** (m) moon
**Shyamala** (m) dark blue
**Sukhadaa** (f) one who brings pleasure
**Suprateekaa** (f) well-proportioned
**Suprabhaa** (f) brilliant
**Supriya** (m/f) greatly liked
**Subaalaa** (f) beautiful maiden
**Suryamukhi** (f) bright as the sun
**Swachland** (f) self-willed
**Swapnila** (f) dreamy
**Sutapa** (m) one who practices austere penances
**Sutapaa** (f)
**Suneela/Sunil** (m) very black, dark blue

# T

**Taralitaa** (f) shaking, undulating
**Tamasvinee** (f) night
**Tami** (f) dark half of the month
**Tandraa** (f) fatigue
**Tanmaya** (m) engrossed
**Tannavee** (f) young
**Tantipaala** (m) cowherd
**Tanujaa** (f) born from body; daughter
**Tapana** (m) sun; summer
**Tapas** (m) heat, penance
**Tapaswinee** (f) one who does penance **Tapasvee** (m)
**Taaraa** (f) a star or planet
**Taaraachand** (m) silver star
**Taaraka** (m) a star, pupil of the eye
**Taralaa** (f) unsteady; splendid
**Tarana** (m) a raft; heaven
**Taranga** (m) wave
**Taranginee** (f) a river
**Taranee** (f) a ray of light; a boat
**Taraswinee** (f) swift; strong
**Taarikaa** (f) beautiful; a small star
**Taarinee** (f) a raft; one who saves others
**Taritree** (f) that which swims; a boat
**Tarlikaa** (f) shaking
**Tarpanaa** (f) pleasing
**Tarulataa** (f) a creeper
**Taruna** (m) youth
**Tarunikaa** (f) young
**Tasmin** (m) literally, 'in that'

**Tavaachaarya** (m) preceptor
**Tatini** (f) a river
**Teekshnaa** (f) sharp-witted
**Teekshnapushpaa** (f) flower of the clove tree
**Teekshnarashmi** (m) the sun
**Tejaa** (m) lustrous
**Tejala** (f) full of light
**Tejas** (m) sharpness
**Tejashree** (f) beauty of the lustre
**Tejasee** (f) lustre
**Tejaswinee** (f) one who has dignity
**Tejni** (f) the edge of a knife; a reed
**Tejapaal** (m) protector of lustre
**Tejaprakaasha** (m) powerful light
**Tilaka** (m) mark made with sandalwood or unguent
**Teertha** (m) holy place
**Teerthaa** (f)
**Titikshaa** (f) endurance
**Tittiri** (m) a partridge
**Timin** (m) a large fish
**Timingila** (m) swallower of the Timin
**Tosha** (f) delighted
**Toshaka** (m) one who pleases
**Toshitaa** (f) satisfied
**Toshala** (f) one who satisfies
**Trapa** (f) modesty
**Trilochanaa** (f) one with three eyes **Trilochana** (m)
**Tribhuvana** (m) three worlds
**Trilokhee** (f) the universe

**Triloka/Tarlok** (m) three worlds

**Tripura** (m) a collection of three cities

**Tripuramba** (f) mother of the three worlds

**Tripuraari** (m) enemy of the three cities

**Triptaa/Truptaa** (f) satisfied

**Tripti/Trupti** (f) satisfaction

**Trushaa** (f) thirst

**Trushitaa** (f) one who desires gain

**Trushnaa** (f) strong desire

**Tuhina** (m) cold

**Tryambaka** (m) three-eyed; or having three wives or sisters

**Tulasi** (f) basil plant

**Tulsidaasa** (m) servant of tulsi

**Tungara** (m) high, lofty

**Tungee** (f) night

**Tungesha** (m) the moon

**Tureeya** (m) the fourth state of the soul

**Tushaara** (m) cold, frosty

**Tushti** (f) satisfaction

**Tvashta** (m) a carpenter

**Twishaa/Twishi** (f) lustrous

**Twesha** (m) bright

**Taralaa** (f) tremulous

**Taralitaa** (f) shaking

**Taaraka** (m) protecting, a star

**Titikshaa** (f) patience

**Tulikaa** (f) brush

# U

Uchitaa (f) appropriate

Udadhi (m) the sea

Ugagra (m) high peak; in the forefront

Udaya (m) to rise

Udayamaana (m) going upwards; accomplishment

Udeepa (m) flood

Udaatta (m) generous

Uddipaka (m) one who stimulates, excites

Uddipta (m) lighted, stimulated Uddipti (f)

Udgata (m) one who sings aloud mantras to summon the deity

Udeit (f) in which the sun rises

Udhyoti (m) the sun

Ugraa (f) fierce Ugra (m)

Ugrayaayi (m) one who walks fiercely

Udyaana (m) park

Ugraayudha (m) one whose weapons are fearful

Ujaas (m) light

Ujesha (m) one who gives light

Ujilaa (f) pure, bright

Ujjalaa (f) one who is bright and beautiful

Ukti (f) speech

Ulkaa (f) a fiery phenomenon

Udita (m) grown; awakened; shining Uditaa (f)

Umaasee (m/f) generous

Ulhaasa (m) joy, delight

Ulhasinee (f) one who is always cheerful

Ulmukha (m) curious, anxious

Umadaa (m) best

Umanga (m) enthusiasm, happiness

Ummesha (m) flash

Umeda (m) hope, wish

Unmilana (m) to be awakened, expanding

Unmukha (m) expectant

Unnati (f) elevation

Unmesha (m) blowing, opening

Upagnaa (f) one with intimate knowledge of

Upaasi (m) a devotee who is offering prayers; one who is fasting

Upaasana (f) attendance, worship

Oorjaa (f) shakti

Oorjashree (f) energy

Oorjasvitaa/Urjaswatee (f) powerful

Oormi (f) waves of emotion, speed

Oormikaa (f) wave; regret; the humming of a bee

Oormila (m) sentimental

Oornaa (f) wool

Oormya (f) night

Ooru (f) thigh

Uru (f) big, expensive

Uruchakshaa (f) with big eyes

Urvee (f) wide region; earth

Urvijaa (f) born of the earth

Urvijayaa (f) victory over the world

Usha (f) dawn

Ushas (f) the dawn

**Ushaakirana** (f) the first light of the dawn

**Usheetaa** (f) one who dwells

**Ushmaa** (f) warmth; anger

**Ushnaa** (f) the hot season

**Utkalikaa** (f) seductive

**Utkarsha** (m) awakening; prosperity

**Utkrushta** (m) best

**Utpala** (m) fleshless; water lily **Utpalaa** (f)

**Utpalaakshee** (f) lotus-eyed

**Utsanga** (m) embrace

**Utsarga** (m) to give up self; pouring out; a gift

**Utsuka** (m) anxiously desirous

**Uttama** (m) best **Uttamaa** (f)

**Utthaana** (m) to arise

**Upaasanaa** (f) worship, service

**Uttaanbarhi** (m) a bird on stretched wings

**Utprekshaa** (f) imagination

**Uttunga** (m) high, lofty

**Urmikaa** (f) ring

**Ushaprabha** (f) light of dawn

# V

Vaachaspati (m) lord of speech
Vaachyaa (f) expressed
Vaageshwaree (f) goddess of
   speech
Vaagheshwaree (f) goddess
   who rides on a tiger
Vaagminee (f) skilful in speech
Vaagminn (m)
Vaibhava (m) one who is rich
   in himself Vaibhavi (f)
Vaidyanaatha (m) scholar
Vaihaayas (m) aerial
Vaihaayasi (f)
Vaijayantee (f) a banner
Vaijayanteekaa (f) a banner;
   a garland of pearls
Vaishwaanara (m) omnipresent
Vaishwaanaree (f)
Vetravatee (f) door-keeper
Vaikuntha (m) holy basil
Vaakpati (m) eloquent
Varun (m) presiding deity
   of water; planet neptune
Vajramani (m) a diamond
Vajraanga (m) diamond-bodied
Vaak (f) speech
Vamshalakshmi (f) the fortune
   of a family
Valaaka (m) a crane
Vallabha (m) beloved, dear
Vallabhee (f)
Vallabhadaas (m) literally,
   dear servant
Vallee (f) a creeper
Vallaree (f) a creeper
Vallakee (f) stringed instrument
Vaalmeeki (m) from Nalmika
   an ant-hill

Vaamaa (f) beautiful
Vaamana (m) short in stature
Vaamaakshee (f) having
   beautiful eyes
Vanadevee (f) goddess of the
   woods
Vanadurgaa (f) goddess of the
   forest
Vanajaa (f) vana = forest;
   jaa = born to
Vanajyoti (f) light of the
   woods
Vanajyotsanaa (f) moonlight
   in the forest
Vanalakshmee (f) the beauty
   of the forest
Vanalataa (f) forest creeper
Vanaalikaa (f) a sun-flower
Vanamaalikaa (f) wood sprite
Vanapriyaa (f) beloved of the
   woods; the koel bird
Vanaraaja (m) king of the
   jungle; the lion
Vanasarojinee (f) the wild
   cotton plant
Vanashree (f) beauty or
   wealth of the woods
Vaanee (f) sound, speech
Vanshidhara (m) a flute-player
Vandana (m) salutation
Vandanaa (f)
Vandanee (f) worship
Vandaneeyaa (f) to be saluted
Vanikaa (f) a little wood
Vanitaa (f) a woman, wife
Vanditaa (f) one praised by
   others
Vapusha (f) a god, deity

**Vaangamati** (f) intelligent in speech

**Varatanu** (f) fair-limbed; beautiful

**Varadaa** (f) bestower of boons

**Varaanganaa** (f) a lovely woman

**Vapaa** (f) a mound of earth thrown up by ants

**Varadaraaja** (m) bestower of boons

**Varaangi** (f) one having a beautiful body

**Varapradaa** (f) one who grants a boon

**Varinee** (f) a woman

**Varnanaa** (f) description

**Varnamaalaa** (f) the alphabet

**Varshaa** (f) shower of rain

**Varchaa** (f) energy, power

**Vareeyans** (m) most excellent

**Varishaa** (f) rain

**Varnikaa** (f) the mask or dress of an actor

**Varshitaa** (f) rained

**Vasudhaa** (f) the earth

**Vageesha** (m) an orator

**Vasanta** (m) spring

**Vasantaa** (f)

**Vasantakumaara** (m) youth

**Varninee** (f) belonging to any one of the four principal castes

**Vaasantee** (f) youthful

**Vasu** (m) wealth

**Vasumat** (m) wealthy, rich

**Vasumati** (f) the earth

**Vasundharaa** (f) the earth

**Vasushree** (m) beauty of wealth

**Vasuttama** (m) grand wealth

**Vatsaadevi** (f) young girl

**Vatsalikaa** (f) affectionate

**Vat** an affix added to nouns to show possession; the adjectives would denote 'similarity' and may be translated by 'like' or 'as'

**Vatsara** (m) a year

**Vaayu** (m) god of victory

**Veda** (m) sacred knowledge

**Vedasmriti** (f) memory of the vedas

**Vedaanga** (m) a part of the vedas

**Velaa** (f) time, season

**Venee** (f) braided hair

**Venu** (m) a bamboo; a reed; a flute

**Vi** as a prefix to verbs and nouns it expresses: the reverse of an action, division, distinction, order, arrangement, opposition, intensity, etc.

**Vibhaa** (f) night

**Vibhava** (m) wealth, dignity

**Vibhaavan** (m) discussion

**Vibhaavaree** (f) night; a harlot; talkative

**Vibhaavasu** (m) the sun, the moon

**Vibhu** (m) mighty, supreme

**Vibhuti** (f) power; ashes

**Vignyaapana** (f) a request

**Vidyullataa** (f) a streak of lightning

**Vidhatru** (m) creator

**Vidhaatri** (f)

**Vidhu** (m) the moon

**Vinati** (f) bowing down

**Vinamra** (m)

**Viraaja** (m) resplendent

**Vipalaanand** (m) great joy

**Vidura** (m) wise

**Vidyaacharana** (m) learned

70

**Vidhushi** (f) a scholar
**Vidhwaana** (m)
**Vidyaagauree** (f) goddess of knowledge
**Vidyaadhara** (m) a class of demi-gods or semi-divine beings
**Vidyut** (f) lightning
**Vidyagauri** (f) Vidya knowledge
**Vighneshwara** (m) lord of obstacles
**Vihanginee** (f) one who flies like a bird
**Vidyaaranya** (m) forest of learning
**Vijaya** (m) victory
**Vijayaalakshmee** (f) Lakshmi's wealth
**Vikartana** (m) the sun
**Vikaasinee** (f) opening
**Vikaasa** (m) expanding; to shine
**Vilaasavatee** (f) amorous
**Viraama** (m) rest
**Vishraama** (m) rest
**Vikrama** (m) the sun of valour
**Vikramaarka** (m)
**Vikramendra** (m) king of prowess
**Vikranta** (m) powerful
**Vikraantaa/Vikraanti** (f)
**Vilaasa** (m) graceful movement of play
**Vilaasini** (f)
**Vilochana** (m) the eye
**Vimala** (m) pure **Vimalaa** (f)
**Vimalalakshmi** (f) Lakshmi, the pure
**Vimarsha** (m) discussion, debate
**Vinantikaa** (f) humility

**Vinayaa** (f) humble
**Vinaya** (m) good manners
**Vinitaa** (f) humble, meek
**Vinit** (m)
**Vinoda** (m) happy; full of joy
**Vinodaa** (f)
**Vinodini** (f) one with a fun-loving character
**Vipana** (m) sail, petty trade
**Vipina** (m) jungle, wood
**Viplava** (m) drifting about
**Vipula** (m) large, great
**Vipulaa** (f) the earth
**Viraja** (m) splendour
**Virajaa** (f) one free from lust or passion
**Virala** (m) unobtainable, rare
**Viraata** (m) having giant proportions
**Veera** (m) hero
**Veerbaalaa** (f) courageous young girl
**Virochana** (m) the moon, fire
**Vishakhaa** (f) without a branch
**Vishaala** (m) broad, great
**Vishaalaaksha** (m) large-eyed
**Vishaalaakshi** (f)
**Vishikhaa** (f) arrow; pin
**Vishnu** (m) root, to pervade
**Vishva** (m) the earth; universe
**Vishvam** (m) universal
**Vishwambara** (m) the supreme spirit
**Vishwaasa** (m) faith, trust
**Vishwamitra** (m) friend of the world
**Vishwampa** (m) one who protects the world
**Vishwarupa** (m) omnipresent
**Vivaswat** (m) the sun
**Viveka** (m) judgement
**Vivekini** (f) discriminating

71

**Vivekaananda** (m) joy of discrimination

**Vivitsu** (m) one who wishes to know

**Viyati** (m) a bird

**Virachanaa** (f) arrangement

**Viyogini** (f) one separated from her lover or husband

**Vrataa** (f) one who performs religious acts

**Vrutti** (f) existing

**Vrindaa** (f) the holy basil

**Vrishali** (f) an unmarried girl

**Vyoma** (f) sky

**Vyomaanga** (m) a part of the sky

**Vyomesha** (m) the sun, moon

**Vyomikaa** (f) one who resides in the sky

# Y

**Yaaja** (m) a brahmin of great sanctity

**Yajna** (m) sacrifice

**Yajnadaya** (f) risen from the sacred fire

**Yagnesha** (m) lord of the sacrificial fire

**Yajnaanga** (m) part of a sacrifice

**Yajamaana** (m) one who performs a regular sacrifice and pays for it; owner

**Yami** (f) night

**Yaamini** (f) night

**Yasha** (m) fame, glory

**Yashapaala** (m) one who protects fame

**Yashaschandra** (m) moon of glory

**Yashodhara** (m) one who has been successful in attaining fame **Yashodharaa** (f)

**Yashodhana** (m) rich in fame

**Yashawanta** (m) one who has attained fame or glory

**Yashaskara** (m) glorious

**Yatin** (m) an ascetic

**Yogini** (f) a sorceress

**Yogamaayaa** (f) the magical power of yoga

**Yoshitaa** (f) a woman, a girl

**Yugandhara** (f) the earth, one who bears the yoke of responsibilities

**Yoganidraa** (f) goddess who has the power to send all creation to sleep

**Yogendra/Yogen** (m) lord of yoga

**Yogeshwara** (m) one who has obtained superhuman faculties

**Yaachanaa** (f) an entreaty

**Yojanaa** (f) union, junction

**Yuthikaa** (f) a variety of jasmine

**Yuti** (f) one who unites

**Yuvaraaja** (m) prince; heir apparent

**Yudhishthira** (m) one who is firm in battle

**Yuyutsu** (m) one who desires to fight

# NAMES OF LORD VISHNU
## *(Vishnushasarnams)*

## A

**Aadhaaranilaya** residing on earth

**Aananda** joy

**Aanandee** joyful

**Aashrama** place of rest, abode

**Aaatmayoni** born on his own

**Aavartana** runs the wheels of the universe

**Abhoo** unborn

**Abhipraaya** intention/wish/ desire/opinion belief

**Achala** static

**Achintya** unthinkable

**Achyuta** unchanged

**Adbhuta** wonderful, extra- ordinary

**Adhaataa** one who is not possessed

**Adhishthaanam** support

**Adhokshaja** with lowered eyes

**Adhruta** cannot be held or possessed

**Aditi** free, boundless, entire happy, pious earth, mother of gods

**Adrashya** invisible

**Agraahya** cannot be grasped

**Agraja** born first

**Agranee** leads ahead

**Aha** praise, deviation from custom

**Aja** existing from all eternity, unborn

**Ajita:** unconcquerable

**Akroora:** not cruel

**Akshaya:** undecaying, unfailing

**Akshara:** imperishable

**Aksharam:** imperishable

**Akshobhya:** one who does not get agitated

**Amaanee:** has no pride

**Amaraprabhu:** immortal god

**Ambhonidhi:** unlimited storate of water

**Ameyaatmaa:** possessing an immeasurable soul, magnanimous

**Amita:** cannot be measured

**Amitaashana:** one who eats a lot

**Amitabikrama:** unlimited heroism

**Amogha:** never fails

**Amoorti:** formless, abstract

**Amoortimaana:** formless, unembodies

**Amruta:** eternal

**Amrutaanshoodbhava:** root of the moon with amrut

**Amrutaasha:** one who drinks nectar

**Amrutapa:** one who drinks nectar

**Amrutavapu:** one who has imperishable body

**Amrutyu:** immortal

**Anaadi:** one who does not have beginning

**Anaadinidhana:** one who has no birth or death

**Anaamaya:** without disease

**Anagha:** without sins

**Anala:** fire

**Ananta:** infinite, eternal

**Anantaatmaa:** eternal soul, supreme soul

**Anantajita:** the conqueror of all

**Anantaroopa:** one who has innumerable shapes and forms

**Anantashree:** boundless magnificance

**Anartha:** meaningless

**Anaya:** cannot be led

**Aneesha:** does not have a lord

**Anekamoorti:** several forms

**Anila:** wind

**Animisha:** vigilant, with steadfast gaze, open

**Aniyama:** no settled rule or direction

**Anirdeshyavapu:** invisible, shapeless soul

**Aniruddha:** independent, without obstacles

**Anivinna:** not depressed or fatigued

**Anivartee:** never regresses

**Anivruttaatmaa:** unfulfilled soul

**Annama:** food

**Antaka:** power of end evey being

**Anu:** atom, smallest particle

**Anuthama:** nobody is greater than him

**Anukoola:** conductive, helpful

**Apaannidhi:** water storage

**Aparaajita:** cannot be defeated

**Apramatta:** alert

**Aprameya:** cannot be measured

**Aprameyaatmaa:** the soul which cannot be measured

**Apratiratha:** unrivalled warrior

**Apyaya:** in whom the universe gets lost

**Archita:** respected, honoured

**Archishmaana:** brilliant

**Arha:** reverent

**Arka:** sun

**Aroudra:** not fierce

**Artha:** wealth

**Arvindaaksha:** eyes like blue lotus

**Asankhyeya:** above the numbers

**Asat:** non-existent

**Ashoka:** devoid of grief, sorrow

**Ashwatha:** 'pipal' free

**Ateendra:** better than Indra

**Ateendreya:** above the senses

**Atula:** beyond comparison

**Avidheyaatmaa:** liberated from obstructions

**Avignaataa:** devoid of special knowledge

**Avishishta:** without anything special

**Avyakta:** invisible

**Avyanga:** no physical deformation

**Avyaya:** no physical destruction

**Ayama:** does not die, cannot be controlled

# B

**Babhru:** one who supports

**Bahushiraa:** one who has numerous blood vessels

**Beejamavyayam:** a seed which cannot be destructed

**Bhaanu:** full of light

**Bhaarabhrut:** bears the burden

**Bhaaskaradyuti:** shining like the sun

**Bhaava:** truth, reality, feeling, love, meaning

**Bhaavana:** always thinks about welfare of devotees

**Bhagahaa:** who destroys grandeur

**Bhagawaana:** overlordship, possessing opulence

**Bhaktavatsala:** shows affection to devotees

**Bhartaa:** one who takes care of every need

**Bhayakrut:** creates fear

**Bhayanaashana:** destroyer of fear

**Bhayaapaha:** destroyer of fear

**Bheema:** who creates fear

**Bheemaparaakrama:** one who has terrific power

**Bheshajam:** medicine

**Bhishak:** doctor

**Bhoktaa:** who enjoys/endures/experiences

**Bhojanam:** that which is enjoyed, wealth

**Bhoobhurva:** sovereign

**Bhoogorbha:** the spirit/soul residing in earth

**Bhootaadi:** the supreme spirit

**Bhooridakshina:** great philanthropist

**Bhooshana:** decoration/ornament

**Bhooshaya:** sleeping on the floor

**Bhootabhaavana:** produces & expands every life

**Bhootabhavyabhavat prabhu:** lord of past, present and future

**Bhootamaheshwara:** lord of all animals

**Bhootaatmaa:** one whose soul is purified

**Bhootaavaasa:** residing in all animals

**Bhraajishnu:** shining, bright, resplendent

**Bhrutkrut:** one who looks after every life

**Bhujagottama:** best snake/Ananta Sheshanaaga

**Braahmana:** one who knows brahmana

**Braahmanapriya:** favourite of braahmanas

**Brahma:** the supreme spirit

**Brahmaa:** creator of universe

**Brahmanya:** does welfare by making others bigger

**Brahmavit:** one who knows supreme spirit

**Bruhat:** biggest of all

**Bruhadbhaanu:** holds great light, lustre

**Bruhadroopa:** having extreme form/appearance

76

# C

**Chakragadaadhara:** who holds 'chakra' ie. sharp circular missile and mace

**Chaanooraandhranishoodana:** one who killed a wrestler by name of 'chaanwoor' ie. Shri Krishna

**Chakree:** supreme being, wind

**Chandanaangadee:** one whose body's parts are adorned with sandalwood paste

**Chandraanshu:** having a cool lustre of moon

**Chaturaatmaa:** god emerging in four places

**Chhinasanshaya:** free from doubt

**Chaturastra:** resides in four places

**Chaturbaabu:** has four arms

**Chaturbhaava:** four different emotions

**Chaturbhuja:** has four hands

**Chaturdrashtra:** has four molar teeth

**Chaturgati:** the supreme soul, a tortoise

**Chaturmoorti:** four different forms

**Chaturvedavit:** knows the four vedas

**Chaturvyooha:** god in form of four 'Vyoohas'

# D

**Daamodara:** bound by rope

**Daaruna:** very frightening

**Daashaarha:** 'dasharha kul' in which Krishna was born

**Daksha:** expert, skilful

**Dakshina:** expert, skilful

**Dama:** one who controls

**Damana:** who suppresses all evil thoughts

**Damayitaa:** keeps in control, suppresses

**Danda:** suppress

**Darpada:** who gives pride

**Darpahaa:** who kills pride

**Deeptamoorti:** god who is brilliant and lustrous

**Deva:** lustrous

**Devabrudguru:** giver and protector of knowledge to gods

**Devakeenandana:** son of Devakee

**Devesha:** lord of gods

**Dhaama:** light

**Dhaataa:** one who holds this universe

**Dhananjaya:** who has won plenty of wealth

**Dhaneshwara:** lord of wealth

**Dhanvee:** one who has a bow

**Dhanya:** fortunate, blessed

**Dhanurdhara:** one who has a bow

**Dhanurveda:** veda concerning archery

**Dharaadhara:** one who holds the earth

**Dharmaadhyaksha:** one who presides over 'dharma'

**Dharma:** one who holds all

**Dharmagup:** protector of 'dharma'

**Dharmakrut:** doer of 'dharma'

**Dharmaviduttama:** best among those who know dharma

**Dharmayoopa:** dharma-like pillar

**Dharaneedhara:** who holds earth

**Dharmee:** who adopts 'dharma'

**Dhrutashee:** one who eats ghee

**Dhrutaatmaa:** one who is stable in one's own unique soul

**Dhruva:** motionless

**Dhurya:** one who holds the axis of the earth

**Disha:** direction

**Divispruk:** one who touches light

**Dradha:** firm

**Drapta:** always cheerful

**Dravinaprada:** giver of wealth to devotees

**Duhaswapnanaashana:** destroyer of bad dreams

**Duraagharsha:** one who cannot be repressed

**Duraarihaa:** destroyer of bad intentions

**Duratikrama:** cannot be overtaken

**Duraavaasa:** residence

**Durdhara:** residence

**Durga:** fort

**Durdhara:** can overcome any difficulty

**Durgama:** difficult to comprehend

**Durlabha:** cannot be obtained easily

**Durjaya:** difficult to win

**Durmarshana:** one who cannot tolerate wicked

**Dushkrutihaa:** destroyer of bad deeds

**Dhyutidhara:** possessing light

# E

**Eka:** one and only

**Ekaatmaa:** one (real) soul

**Ekapaat:** happening at once, suddenly

# G

**Gabhastinemi:** having brilliant circumference

**Gabheera:** serious

**Gabheeraatmaa:** immeasurable soul

**Gadaadhara:** one who holds the mace

**Gadaagraja:** one who is ahead of words ie. light

**Gahana:** incomprehensible

**Gatisattama:** the best movement

**Garudadhwaja:** flag with the symbol of eagle

**Ghrutaashee:** one who eats 'ghee' which is a symbol of fragrance and brightness

**Gnnaanagamya:** that which can be achieved through knowledge

**Guru:** great element

**Gurutama:** best among 'gurus'

**Gnaanamuttamam:** best form of knowledge

**Gohita:** welfare of the senses

**Gopati:** lord of senses, speech and earth

**Goptaa:** protector

**Govindaanpati:** lord of those who know speech and other senses

**Govinda:** one who knows the senses, earth, brahman vidya and is protector of cows

**Graamanee:** who leads the five elements

**Guha:** remaining secretly

**Guhya:** secret

**Gunabhrut:** one who holds all the three 'guna'—satva, rajas and tamas

**Gupta:** invisible

# H

**Hansa:** spirit; swan
**Hari:** one who takes away desires
**Halaayudha:** possessing plough as weapon
**Havi:** material for 'yagna'
**Hemaanya:** with body like gold colour

**Hetu:** end objectives
**Hiranyagarbha:** spirit in form of egg/brilliant as gold
**Hrishkesha:** lord of the sense, 'Indriyas'
**Hutabhuk:** who enjoys the offerings given in 'yagna'

# I

**Iijya:** worth revering
**Iishaana:** north-east direction; god
**Iishwara:** one who has unlimited abilities

**Indrakarmaa:** as heroic as Indra
**Ishta:** of one's liking; imaginary

# J

**Jagadaadija:** one who is born first in the world

**Jagatasetu:** like a bridge of the universe

**Jahnu:** one who kills; one who carries

**Jal:** victory

**Janeshwara:** god residing in the hearts of all

**Janmamrutyujaraatiga:** one who has overcome birth, death and old age

**Janajanmaadi:** fundamental cause of birth

**Janana:** creator, father

**Jayanta:** victor

**Janaardana:** one who kills 'asura' traits

**Jeeva:** life

**Jeevana:** life

**Jetaa:** conquerer; victor

**Jitaamitra:** winner of enemies

**Jitakrudha:** one who wins anger

**Jitamanyu:** one who wins anger

**Jyeshtha:** eldest

**Jyoti:** light

**Jyotiraaditya:** brilliant as the sun

**Jyotirganeshwara:** lord of planets

# K

**Ka:** joy, happiness

**Kaala:** time

**Kaalaneminihaa:** one who kills the wheel of time

**Kaama:** desire

**Kaamadeva:** one who fulfils all desires

**Kaamahaa:** one who kills desires

**Kaamakrut:** one who creates desires

**Kaamaprada:** giver of all desires

**Kaamee:** one who controls the desires

**Kaanta:** one with beautiful body

**Kaaraam:** creator of the universe

**Kanakaangadee:** wearing gold bangles

**Kapeendra:** lord of monkeys

**Kapi:** Sun

**Kapila:** a great sage; tawny

**Kartaa:** creator

**Kathita:** one who is praised by everyone

**Kavi:** a seer who can see the truth

**Keshava:** one who has brilliant rays

**Keshihaa:** one who killed 'keshi' demon

**Khandaparashu:** to break into pieces by an axe

**Kim:** what

**Krama:** power, strength

**Kratu:** form of soma yagna

**Krodhahaa:** one who overcomes anger

**Krudhakrutkartaa:** one who creates anger

**Krusha:** minute

**Krushna:** one who attracts

**Krutagna:** one who graciously accepts the action done out of the love for god

**Krutaagama:** creator of 'aagama', vedas

**Krutaantakrut:** visible and invisible

**Krutalakshana:** one who has created characteristics to achieve god

**Kruti:** self motivated action

**Krutakarmaa:** attains all deeds

**Kshama:** capable

**Kshaminaam vara:** best among those who forgive

**Ksharma:** destroyable

**Kshemakrut:** protector of whatever is achieved

**Kshetragna:** 'god' residing in the body

**Kshiteesha:** lord of earth

**Kshobhana:** one who shakes up

**Kumbha:** container

**Kumuda:** white lily

**Kunda:** clean

**Kundalee:** one who possesses ear ornaments

**Kundara:** one who splits the earth

**Kuvaleshya:** god lying on 'Shesha naag'

# L

**Lakshmee:** beauty, lustre

**Lakshmeevaan:** endowed with wealth

**Lohitaaksha:** one with red eyes

**Lokaadhishthaanam:** support of all the people

**Lokaadhyaksha:** presiding over all the worlds/peoples

**Lokabandhu:** friend of all the worlds

**Lokanaatha:** lord of all the worlds

**Lokasaaranga:** one who absorbs the meaning of all the worlds

**Lokatrayaashraya:** supporting three worlds

# M

Maadhava: sweet as honey
Maanadas: one who destroys
  pride, giver of honour
Maanya: one who is revered
  by all
Maarya: proper course
Madhu: sweet honey
Madhusudana: one who killed
  demon 'Madhu'
Mahaabala: great strength
Mahaabhaaga: extremely rich
Mahaabhoga: one who is in
  great happiness
Mahaabuddhi: one with great
  intellect
Mahaadeva: god who is like
  a great light
Mahaadhana: one who is in
  the form of highest riches
Mahaadridhruk: one who is
  holding great mountain
Mahaadyuti: great splendour,
  beauty
Mahaagarta: state of nothing-
  ness; non-existent
Mahaahavi: great materials
  offered as oblation in yagna
Mahaahruda: great lake
Mahaakarmaa: one who does
  great deeds
Mahaakratu: great 'yagna'
Mahaakosha: great cover
Mahaakrama: one whose
  steps are great
Mahaaksha: great seer
Mahaamakha: great yagna
Mahaamanaa: large hearted
Mahaan: great

Mahaanidhi: where all are
  residing
Mahaamorti: great form
Mahaarha: deserving of great
  prayer
Maharddhi: great intellect
Mahaashakti: great power
Mahaashana: one who ab-
  solves everything
Mahaashrunga: with big horns
Mahaasvana: great sound
Mahaatapaa: whose 'tapa' is
  great
Mahaatejaa: great glory
Mahaaveerya: great adventure
Mahaavaraaha: great boar
Mahaayagna: great yagna
Mahaayajwaa: one who
  performs great yagna
Maheebhartaa: protector of
  the earth
Maheedhara: one who holds
  the earth
Mahudadhishaya: one who
  has slept in the ocean
Mahoraga: great serpent
Mahotsaaha: one with great
  enthusiasm
Mangalamparam: the most
  auspicious
Manohara: one who wins the
  heart
Manojova: as speedy as the
  wind
Manu: founder father of
  human beings
Mantra: spell; charm
Mareechi: one who is brilliant

85

**Medhaja:** one who has emerged from yagna

**Medhaavee:** very intelligent, learned

**Medinepati:** lord of earth

**Mukunda:** one who gives freedom

# N

**Naaraayana:** one who resides in five elements

**Naarasinghavapu:** taking the form of Narsinha Yayoti

**Naika:** many, several

**Naikaatma:** one who has several forms

**Naikaja:** several births

**Naikakarmakrut:** one who has been 'kartaa' in several forms

**Naikamaaya:** one who creates illusions

**Naikaroopa:** one who takes many forms

**Naikashrunga:** with several peaks

**Nakshatranemi:** circumscribed by planets

**Nakshatree:** lord of the planets

**Nanda:** having all kinds of achievements

**Nandakee:** sword

**Nandana:** one who gives joy

**Nandi:** great joy

**Nara:** man

**Naya:** one who leads

**Netaa:** leader

**Neya:** one who is led

**Nidhiravyaya:** storage which cannot be reduced

**Nimisha:** one who can see within

**Nigraha:** independent

**Nirguna:** supreme spirit

**Nirvaanam:** emancipation, liberation

**Nishthaa:** faith

**Niruthaatmaa:** free from bondage

**Niyama:** one who keeps within rules

**Niyantaa:** one who regulates

**Nyagrodha:** banyan tree

**Nyaaya:** justice

# O

**Ojastejodhyutidhara:** one who holds light

**Oorjita:** strong, powerful

**Oorjitashaasana:** rule of powerful

# P

aapanaashana: destroyer of sins

aavana: sanctifying

adamanuttamam: having the highest status/position

admagarbha: in the middle of the lotus

admanibhekshana: eyes like lotus

admee: one who holds lotus in the hand

ana: one who transacts the affairs of the universe

aramaatmaa: the great soul/ supreme spirit

aramapashta: very pure and transparent

arameshthee: one residing in best stations

arameshwara: lord of all; supreme lord

ararddhi: one who extends, expands greatly

rigraha: one who accepts offerings

rjanya: rain

ryavasthita: pervasive in all four directions

vana: clean, pure

vitram: sacred, holy

shala: delicate

orna: complete

orayitaa: one who fulfils all wishes

otaatmaa: sacred soul

abhava: lord from whom everything emanates

abhu: lord

Prabhoota: lord who takes birth in highest way

Pradyumna: man of knowledge; son of Krishna

Pragraha: accepting firmly and with sentiments

Praana: life

Praanabhrut: supporter of life

Praanada: giver of life

Praananilaya: where spirit/ soul resides

Prajaabhava: through whom entire progeny is created

Prajagara: who is always awake, alert

Prajaapah: very first creator of all life/animals

Prakaashana: one who illuminates all

Prakaashaatmaa: form of light, lustre

Pramaanam: measure

Pramodana: one who gives joy

Praanshu: high, lofty/ one of great stature

Pranava: the sacred syllable Om

Prasannaatmaa: cheerful soul

Prapitaamaha: one who originated the world

Prataapana: powerful, majestic

Pratardana: one who destructs

Prathita: welknown

Pratishthita: famous, valued

Pratyaya: one who is knowledge itself

**Preetivardhana:** continuously increasing love

**Priyakrut:** who endures

**Priyaarha:** dear and revered

**Pruthu:** large

**Punarvasu:** resides in various bodies over and over again

**Pundareekaaksha:** eyes like lotus

**Punya:** righteous, holy

**Punyakeerti:** holy fame

**Punyashravanakeertana:** auspicious to recite and hear

**Puraatana:** ancient

**Purandara:** one who destroys town

**Purujit:** one who wins affection of all

**Purusha:** the supreme being

**Purusattama:** one who is best in town

**Purushottama:** best among men

**Pushkaraaksha:** lotus like ey

**Pushpahaasa:** smile like full blown flower

**Pushta:** perfected

# R

**Raama:** pleasing, charming

**Rakshana:** protection

**Ranapriya:** one who loves battlefield

**Ratnagarbha:** heart is brilliant like jewel

**Rathaangapaani:** one who holds the wheel of chariot

**Ravi:** sun

**Ravilochana:** eyes like the sun

**Rohita:** red coloured

**Ruchiraangada:** has beautiful armlets

**Ruddha:** possessed of wealth

**Rutu:** wheel of time/season

# S

**Saadhu:** 'saatvika' man

**Saakshee:** a seer who can see beyond

**Saama;** always same/'saama' veda

**Saamaga:** knows 'saama' veda

**Saamagaayana:** one who sings 'saama' hymns

**Saatvatanpati:** lord of saatvataa's — those who were born in 'Dashaarha' family are also called saatvataa

**Saattvika:** possessed of 'sathva' quality which included calm, peaceful, truthful, honest, virtuous, strong, vigorous

**Sadaamarshee:** always tolerant

**Sadaayogee:** always a yogee

**Sabhooti:** divine, superhuman

**Sadgati:** takes the right path

**Saha:** one who tolerates

**Sahastrajit:** victory of thousands

**Sahasramoordhhaa:** with thousand hands

**Sahasraanshu:** with thousand rays

**Sahasraakshu:** with thousand eyes

**Sahasraarchi:** with thousand rays

**Sahasrapaat:** with thousand feet

**Sahishnu:** who tolerates everything

**Sama:** one who is always same

**Samaatmaa:** who is equal among all living beings

**Samavarta:** who revolves the universe properly

**Samayagna:** who has knowledge of five 'kaals'

**Sambhava:** evenly moving wind

**Sameehana:** wishful, with wishes

**Samitijaya:** one who gets victory in assembly or battle

**Sammita:** one who is encircled equally

**Sampramardana:** able to suppress well

**Sanaat:** eternal

**Sanaatanatama:** eternal

**Santa:** one who has element of 'sat', truth

**Sandhaataa:** one who unites

**Sandhimaan:** soul which is united

**Sangraha:** one who stores what is necessary to restart the world after its destruction/collection

**Sankarshanochyuta:** totally and simultaneously attracts

**Sanksheptaa:** abridged, short

**Sannivaasa:** one who resides in the heart of devotees who follow truth

**Sansthaana:** the soul which has forms and organs

**Sanvruta:** covered

**Saptajihya:** one with seven tongues, ie. with fire

**Sansyaasakruta:** one who liberates from all worthy attachments

**Sanvatsara:** a year — the time earth takes to revolve around sun — one with which season starts

**Saptaidhaa:** one who consumes seven elements in order to unite with divine soul

**Saptavaahana:** one who has a vehicle of sun with seven horses

**Sarga:** Universe which is his creation

**Sarva:** one who includes everything/everyone

**Sarvaadi:** fundamental cause of all

**Sarvaasunilaya:** residence of all soul

**Sarvadarshana:** one who sees everything

**Sarvadarshee:** one who sees all

**Sarvadrugvyaasa:** seeing everyone clearly

**Sarvadruk:** one who observes all

**Sarvaga:** one who can go everywhere

**Sarvavageshwareshwara:** lord of all the speeches

**Sarvagna:** one who knows all/everything

**Sarvakaamada:** one who fulfils all the wishes

**Sarvalakshnaalakshanya:** one who is understood/known by using all the characteristics/qualities

**Sarvasaha:** one who can tolerate everything

**Sarvapraharanaayudha:** all the instruments that can attack are his weapons

**Sarvashastrabhurutaanvara:** one who holds all weapon and knows the best use of

**Sarvatashchakshu:** one who sees all

**Sarvatomukha:** one who has face towards everybody

**Sarvavaageeshwareshwara:** lord of all speech

**Sarvavidbhaanu:** one who knows everything and is lustorous

**Sarvavijjayee:** one who has won all

**Sarvayogavinissruta:** one who has gone through all yoga in a special manner

**Sarveshwara:** lord of all

**Sat:** truth

**Sataangati:** movement of 'satpurusha'

**Satkartaa:** one who creates truth

**Satkeerit:** famous

**Satkruta:** one through whom a good deed is done

**Satkruti:** beautiful creation

**Satparaayanam:** eternally truthful life

**Satpathaachaara:** follower of right path

**Satram:** duration between beginning and end of 'yagna'

**Sattaa:** power

**Sattvastha:** residing in pure element

**Sattvavaan:** virtuous

**Saatvika:** endowed with the quality of sattva ie goodne

**Satya:** truth

**Satyadharmaa:** one whose dharma is truth

**Satyadharmaparaakrama:** one whose valour has truth and 'dharma'

**Satyadharmaparaayana:** one who is absorbed in truth and duty

**Satyamedhaa:** intellect involved in truth

**Satyaparaakrama:** one who performs truthful adventures

**Satyaparaayanam:** one who is solely devoted to truth

**Sava:** 'somayagna'

**Savitaa:** sun

**Shaanta:** peace

**Shaanti:** peace

**Shaantida:** giver of peace

**Shaarngadhanvaa:** one who holds 'shaarng' bow

**Shaashwata:** indestructible

**Shashwatasthaanu:** always immovable

**Shashwatasthira:** always immovable

**Shaastaa:** one who rules

**Shabdaatiga:** one who is above words

**Shaktimataanshreshtha:** best among powerful

**Shama:** forgiveness

**Shambhu:** one who gives peace, happiness & welfare

**Shankhabhrut:** one who holds conch shell

**Sharabha:** an imagined 'puranic' animal, who could kill lion

**Sharanam:** last resort

**Sharirabhrut:** one who nurtures body

**Sharma:** blessings, protection

**Shataananda:** unlimited happiness

**Sharva:** one who can kill everything. This is the name of Shiva but by including it in 'Vishnusahstranaama' the unity between Shiva and Vishnu is shown

**Sharvareekara:** creator of 'great night' ie. when body sleeps but soul and its power is awake

**Shashabindu:** one who has sign of rabbit ie. moon

**Shataanana:** having several faces

**Shataavarta:** one who has several incarnations

**Shatamoorti:** having several forms

**Shatrughna:** one who kills enemies

**Shatrunjita:** victory over enemies

**Shatrutaapana:** one who agitates enemies

**Shipivishta:** one who resides in animals

**Shishira:** name of a season

**Shishtakrut:** one who does honourable deeds

**Shishteshta:** desired by proper learned people

**Shiva:** one who does welfare

**Shokanaashana:** one who destroys sorrow

**Shoonya:** zero/nothing

**Shoora:** very adventurous

**Shoorajaneshwara:** lord of heroes

**Shraman:** one who performs penance

**Shoorasena/Shouri:** one who is born in 'shoora' family, i.e. Vasudeva's

**Shreshtha:** best among all

**Shreya:** great prosperity/welfare

**Shreeda:** giver of wealth, Laxmi

**Shreedhara:** one who holds 'Laxmi' in heart

**Shreegarbha:** one in whose heart Laxmi resides

**Shreekara:** one who raises the divine attributes (Shri means attributes such as fame, speech, praise, intelligence, forgiveness)

**Shreemaan:** one who has wealth

**Shreenidhi:** store of wealth

**Shreenivaasa:** in whose heart 'Laxmi' wealth resides

**Shreepati:** lord of 'Laxmi'

**Shreesha:** lord of wealth

**Shreevaasa:** where 'Laxmi' is residing

**Shreevatsavakshaa:** possessing the sign of affection on chest

**Shreevibhaavana:** distributing wealth as on deserve

**Shrungee:** incarnation of god in form of fish with horns

**Shrutisaagara:** storage of Vedas

**Shubhaanga:** who has nice parts of the body

**Shubhekshana:** auspicious sight 'Drasthi'

**Shuchi:** sacred, holy

**Shuchishravaa:** one who is 'pavitra', sacred to listen to

**Siddhi:** achieving fullness

**Siddha:** one who has attained supernatural powers

**Siddhaartha:** one who has acquired all 'siddhis'

**Siddhasankalpa:** one who determination is complete

**Siddhida:** giver of 'siddhis'

**Siddhisaadhana:** one who helps to achieve 'siddhis'

**Sinha:** all powerful, heroic

**Skanda:** one who leaps out, divine power

**Skandadhara:** one who holds divine power

**Soma:** one who showers nectar

**Somapa:** one who drinks 'soma'

**Sookshma:** minute, very small

**Soorya:** sun

**Spashtaakshara:** distinct/evident supreme being

**Sragvee:** one who wears necklace

**Srashtaa:** creator of universe

**Stavapriya:** one who likes the praise

**Stavya:** worth praising

**Sthaanu:** one who is always immovable

**Sthaanadu:** one who gives position

**Sthavira Dhruva:** very ancient and immovable

**Sthavishtha:** huge form

**Sthira:** immovable

**Sthoola:** gross/material/bulky

**Stotaa:** one who sings praise adulation

**Stotram:** hymn of praise

**Stuti:** hymn of praise

**Subhuja:** with beautiful arms

**Sudarshana:** beautiful looks

**Sudhanvaa:** possessing best bow

**Sughosha:** one who makes beautiful sound

**Suhruta:** great friend residing in all animals

**Sukhada:** one who gives happiness

**Sulabha:** easily available

**Sulochana:** beautiful eyes

**Sumedhaa:** fine intellect

**Sumukha:** beautiful face

**Sunda:** merciful, compassionate

**Sundara:** beautiful

**Suparna:** with beautiful wings

**Suprasaada:** very generous

**Suraananda:** one who gives pleasure to gods

**Suraarihaa:** one who destroys the enemies of god

**Suresh:** lord of gods

**Sureshwara:** lord of lustrous gods

**Suruchi:** very beautiful/likeable

**Sushena:** army in form of heavenly riches

**Sutantu:** one who is like a thread of love and beauty

**Sutapaa:** one who performs great penance

**Suvarnabindu:** gold like drop/point

**Suvarnavarna:** colour of skin as lustrous as gold

**Suveera:** beautifully moving

**Suvrata:** one who is discipline

**Suyamuna:** residing on the banks of river 'Yamuna' ie. Shri Krishna

**Swaapana:** one who can give up all the dreams

**Swaabhaavya:** one who can be born on his own

**Swaasya:** beautiful face

**Swadhruta:** one who holds himself

**Swaksha:** beautiful and adorned eyes

**Swanga:** beautiful parts of body

**Swaanga:** guise/personation

**Swasti:** benediction

**Swastibhook:** one who experiences benediction

**Swastida:** one who looks after welfare

**Swastidakshina:** one who is always anxious and generous to give benediction

**Swastikrut:** one who does good for all

**Swavasha:** master of oneself

**Swayambhoo:** one who is born of himself

**Swayamjaata:** one who is born on his own

# T

**Taara:** best sound
**Taarana:** one who uplifts
**Tantuvardhana:** keeps expanding the fibre
**Tat:** consequently/for that reason/therefore
**Tattravam:** essence
**Tattvavit:** one who knows the essence
**Tejovrusha:** one who showers light
**Teerthakara:** creator of 'tirtha'
**Tridarshaadhyaksha:** lord of 3 stages, (awakened, semi awakened and sleep)

**Trikakubdhadhaama:** a resting place of all the three directions (high, middle and low) in which the soul travels
**Trilokadhruk:** holding 3 worlds
**Trilokaatmaa:** soul of the 3 worlds
**Trilokesha:** lord of 3 worlds
**Trisaamaa:** one who is praised by 3 notes and 3 scales
**Trivikrama:** Vishnu in fifth/ dwarf incarnation
**Tushta:** contented
**Tvashtaa:** one who arranges, constructs

# U

**Udbhava:** source, origin, birth
**Udeerna:** best
**Udumbara:** name of a tree
**Ugra:** powerful
**Upendra:** close to Indra
**Urdhwaga:** moving upwards

**Urjita:** great valour, heroism
**Urjitashaasana:** regulator of ascending power
**Uttara:** highest form
**Uttaarana:** one who rescues

# V

**Vaachaspati:** the lord of speech

**Vaagmee:** lord of speech

**Vaamana:** dwarf

**Vaaruna:** name of god

**Vaasavaanuja:** Indra's younger brother Upendra

**Vaasudeva:** one who resides in all

**Vaayu:** wind

**Vaayuvaahana:** carrier of wind

**Vahni:** a god

**Vaidya:** has all types of knowledge

**Vaikhaana:** one who digs in a special manner

**Vaikuntha:** heavenly abode of Vishnu/paradise

**Vanamaalee:** one who wears 'Vaijayanti' garland

**Vanshavardhana:** who expands 'Vansha' family

**Varada:** gives blessings

**Varaanga:** best body

**Varaaroha:** having highest status

**Vardhana:** giver of property

**Vardhamaana:** who has prospered

**Vashatkaara:** one who is offered sacrifice

**Vasu:** one who dwells in all

**Vasuda:** giver of 'saatvik' revelation

**Vasumanaa:** with a rich heart

**Vasuprada:** giver of pure lustre

**Vasuretaa:** shining like gold

**Vatsala:** affectionate, kind

**Vatsara:** year

**Vatsee:** looking after devotees affectionately

**Veda:** a kind of holy scripture

**Vedavit:** who knows 'Vedas'

**Vedaanga:** 'Veda' is a part of him

**Vedhaa:** creator of the universe

**Vedya:** worth knowing

**Veera:** hero

**Veerabaahu:** with heroic arms

**Veerahaa:** one who destroys heroes

**Veetabhaya:** fearless

**Vegavaan:** very speedy

**Vibhu:** all pervasive

**Vidaarana:** destroyer

**Vidhaataa:** possessing several forms

**Vidhwatthama:** best among the learned

**Vidisha:** regulates directions and corners

**Vijaya:** victor

**Vijitaatmaa:** victorious soul

**Vihaayasagati:** moving in the sky, bird

**Vikrama:** one who can overcome all

**Vikramee:** victor, great adventurer

**Vikshara:** devoid of annihilation

**Vimuktaatmaa:** always free

**Viraama:** rest

**Vinaya:** one who follows rules

**Vinayitaasaakshee:** witness to politeness

**Virata:** devoid of attachment

**Virochana:** one who creates special liking

**Vishama:** hard to understand/ very strong

**Vishwam:** universe

**Visihishta:** one who is special

**Vishnu:** all pervasive god

**Vishodhana:** one who finds the soul of the self

**Vishoka:** without sorrow

**Vishraama:** rest

**Vishrutaatmaa:** whose fame is spread in extraordinary way

**Vishuddhaatmaa:** pure soul

**Vishwabaahu:** helps support the universe

**Vishwabhuk:** who enjoys the universe

**Vishwadakshina:** expert of the universe

**Vishwadhruk:** who holds the universe

**Vishwakarmaa:** architect of the universe

**Vishvaksena:** no army can overcome him

**Vishwamoorti:** one in form of universe

**Vivikta:** resides in solitude

**Vishwaatmaa:** soul of the universe

**Vishwayoni:** place from where universe was born

**Vistaara:** pervasive, expansion

**Vruddhaatmaa:** most ancient soul

**Vrushaakapi:** an epithet of Vishnu

**Vruksha:** one who showers, rain, light, pleasure etc.

**Vrushabha:** anything best or eminent of its class

**Vrushabhaaksha:** one with righteous approach

**Vrushkarmaa:** whose deeds are like 'Dharma'

**Vrushaakruti:** who is actual form of 'Dharma'

**Vrushaparvaa:** who is like steps of 'Dharma'

**Vrushapriya:** who loves to be rightesous

**Vyaadisha:** who gives special orders — regulates universe

**Vyagra:** busy, worried

**Vyaktaroopa:** visible

**Vyaala:** a king

**Vyaapee:** all pervading

**Vyavasaaya:** occupation

**Vyavasthaana:** who arranges the universe

# Y

**Yadushreshtha:** best among yadus

**Yagna:** sacrifice/any oblation/ an act of worship

**Yagnabhuk:** who gets the fruits of yoga

**Yagbhut:** holding sacrificai rites

**Yagnaguhyam:** secret of yagna (worship)

**Yagnakrut:** performer of sacrifice, offering

**Yagnaanga:** ports of yagna (sacrifice)

**Yagnapati:** lord of yagna (sacrifice)

**Yagnasaadhana:** procured through yagna (oblation)

**Yagnavaahana:** one who carries 'yagna', oblation

**Yagnee:** who accepts sacri- ficial rites

**Yajwaa:** performer of sacrifice

**Yama:** controlling/any great moral or religious duty

**Yat:** to strive after/be watch- ful/to long for

**Yoga:** way of becoming one with god

**Yogavidaam Netaa:** the leader who knows how to be one with god

**Yogee:** one who follows, the philosophy/way of be- coming one with god

**Yogeesha:** one who has bo- tained superhuman faculties

**Yugaadikrut:** one who started the eras

**Yugaavarta:** one who changes all the eras

# NAMES OF LORD SHIVA
## *(Shivashasarnams)*

## A

**Aaloka:** splendour, light, a word of praise uttered by a bard

**Aamnaaya:** like veda

**Aananda:** joy

**Aashrama:** one giving tranquility like aashrama

**Aatmabhoo:** self generated

**Aatmajyoti:** brilliant on his own or through his own soul

**Aatmayoni:** self created

**Aayushabdapati:** lord of duration of life and words

**Abhava:** without birth

**Abheda:** undivided, identical

**Abheeru:** fearless

**Abhiraama:** pleasing, delightful, beautiful

**Abhichaaryo Mahaamaya:** one who creates great illusions

**Achala:** steady, immovable

**Achaleshwara:** lord of immovable world

**Achanchala:** steady, immovable

**Achintya:** inconceivable

**Adeena:** one who is not poor or not distressed or not dejected or not frightened

**Adharmashatru:** destroyer of unrighteousness, injustice or enemy of injustice

**Adhokshaja:** incomprehensible by sense organ

**Adhoorta:** one who is not cunning

**Adhruta:** without any support or one who does not need support

**Adhyaatmayoganilaya:** where spiritualism and yoga resides

**Adrayaalaya:** residing on mountain

**Adri:** like mountain

**Agastya:** like Agastya, who was a sage

**Aghora:** not fierce

**Agneya:** impossible to know

**Agraha:** difficult to comprehend

**Aguna:** a fault or without virtues

**Aha:** day

**Aharpati:** like sun

**Ahankaara:** pride

**Aishwaryajanmamrityujaraatiga:** one who is without birth, death or old age because of divinity

**Aja:** unborn i.e. existing from all eternity

**Ajaatashatru:** one who does not have any enemy or one who does not lose out to an enemy

**Ajitapriya:** the loved one who is invincible

**Akaala:** timeless

**Akalmasha:** without sin or without blemish

**Akampa:** steady

**Akampita:** immovable, steady

**Akshayaguna:** who has eternal virtues

**Akshunna:** who cannot be insulted

**Alankarishnu:** who ornates all

**Alobha:** without greed

**Amoghadanda:** the mark of whose mace never fails

**Amoghorishtanemi:** who destroys enemies with never failing axle of the wheel i.e. a heavenly body

**Amrutaansha:** nectar is a part of him

**Amrutamaya:** like nectar or in the form of nectar

**Amrutapa:** who drinks nectar

**Amruta shaashwata:** immortal as nectar

**Amrutavapu:** whose body is immortal

**Amrutyu:** without death

**Anaadi:** without beginning

**Anaadimadhyanidhana:** without beginning, interim and end

**Anaadyanta:** without beginning and end

**Anaamaya:** healthy, free from disease

**Anagha:** faultless

**Ananta:** without an end

**Anapaayokshara:** indestructable and eternal

**Anartha:** without purpose

**Anarthita:** who does not beg

**Anarthanaashana:** who destroys misunderstandings, misconceptions

**Andhakaaree:** enemy of a demon by name of Andhaka

**Anekakrut:** having many forms

**Angiraa:** like Angira sage who received the 'Brahmavidya' from Atharvan and imparted it to Satyavaha

**Anirdeshyavayu:** with invisible body

**Aniruddha:** uncontrolled, free

**Anivaarita:** who cannot be restricted

**Aniyama:** one who is above rules

**Anu:** very little or smallest part of time

**Anuttamo duraagharsha:** nobody is better than him and he who is not defeated by anybody

**Anuttara:** the best

**Apaannidhi:** like an ocean

**Aparaajita:** unconquerable

**Aparichhedya:** one who cannot be measured with time and place

**Apratimaakruti:** exceptional form

**Araaga:** without anger

**Arindama:** destroyer of enemies

**Artha:** meaning, significance

**Arthada:** one who gives wealth

**Arthavichchhambhu:** one who knows vedas and does welfare

**Asaadhya:** unobtainable

**Asansrushta:** not connected

**Arthigamya:** one who should be worshipped by those who wish to go to heaven

**Asankhyeyoprameyaatmaa:** who cannot be counted or measured

**Ashtamoorti:** one who is an embodiment of eight elements viz sky, water, fire, wind, earth, sun, moon and soul

**Asuavyaaghra:** like a tiger for demons

**Ateendriyo mahaamaya:** great illusory who is above senses

**Atithi:** guest

**Atri:** like sage Atri, author of many vedic hymns

**Avaangamanasagochara:** one who cannot be understood or comprehended by speech or mind

**Avyakta Lakshano Deva:** god who is not visible but can be perceived

**Avyaya:** imperishable or immutable

# B

**Baalroopa:** in the form of child (one who was born in the form of child)

**Baanaadhyaksha:** presiding over sound or voice

**Baanahasta prataapavaan:** the powerful, majestic one holding the arrow in hand

**Badhira:** deaf

**Bahuroopa:** with many forms

**Bahushruti:** one who has given several 'shrutis'

**Balanidhi:** store of force, power

**Balavaan:** powerful

**Balee:** powerful

**Balonmatta:** intoxicated with strength, power

**Beejavaahana:** who carried seed (truth)

**Beejakartaa:** creator of seed of the world

**Bhaalnetra:** who has an eye on the forehead

**Bhaanu:** sun

**Bhaavaatmaatmani Sansthita:** residing in every soul with love, affection

**Bhaganetrabhit:** destroyer of 'Bhaga's' eyes

**Bhagawaana:** divinity, over-lordship

**Bhagovivasvaanaaditiyo:** who is like sun

**Bhaktalokadhruk:** who holds the group of devotees

**Bhakikaaya:** devotion personified

**Bhasmapriyao Bhasmashaayee:** who loves ashes and sleeps on ashes

**Bhasmashuddhikara:** purifies with ashes

**Bhasmodhullita Vigraha:** who has ashes all over the body

**Bhavya:** the best

**Bhima:** fierce, formidable

**Bhima paraakrama:** with formidable acts

**Bhishak:** like a physician

**Bhojanam:** meals

**Bhoktaa:** one who enjoys experiences

**Bhoobhurvo Laxmi:** one who adorn the earth and heaven

**Bhoodeva:** god on earth or Brahmin

**Bhoopati:** lord of earth

**Bhooshana:** ornament

**Bhooshaya:** who sleeps on floor

**Bhootabhaavana:** increasing, expanding the number of lives

**Bhoota Bhavya Bhavannaatha:** lord of past, present and future

**Bhootakrut:** creator of every creature

**Bhootapaala:** protector of everyone

**Bhootasatyaparaayana:** supporter of the living beings

**Bhootavaahana:** carrier of every being

**Bhraajishnu:** lustrous

**Bhooti:** who was material-
istic wealth

**Bhootinaashana:** destroyer of
enemy's property

**Bhrutyamarkataroopadhruk:**
becoming a servant in the
form of Haruman

**Bindu Sanshraya:** in form
of 'Om'

**Braahmana:** a priest, also an
epithet of 'Agni' (fire)

**Braahmanapriya:** who is loved
by priests

**Brahmaa:** like Brahmaa,
creator of the world

**Brahmaandahrut:** destroyer of
the universe

**Brahmachaaree:** who moves
about in the universe

**Brahmagarha:** in whom there
are vedas/universe

**Brahmajyoti:** having Brahma
like light

**Brahmasruk:** creator of
Brahmaa

**Brahmavarchasva:** having
power, lustre like Brahmaa

**Brahmavedanidhi:** storehouse
Brahma and Veda

**Bruhadashva:** who has a
chariot with big horses

**Bruhadgarbha:** who has
Brahman inside

**Budha:** who knows everything

# C

**Chanda:** dreadful, angry

**Chandra:** moon

**Chandramoulee:** who has
moon on head

**Chandrapeeda:** who has moon
as a crown

**Chandrasanjeevana:** giving life
to moon

**Charaachara;** animate and
inanimate i.e. whole world

**Charaacharagra:** who knows
animate and inanimate i.e.
the universe

**Charuvishalya:** beautiful and
without pain

**Chaturbaahu:** with four arms

**Chaturaschaturapriya:** who
likes clever, smart

**Chaturbhaava:** your dis-
positions of mind

**Chaturmukha:** with four faces

**Chaturveda:** like for vedas

**Chatushpatha:** who is like
four roads, such as reli-
gion, wealth, desires and
emancipation

**Chhinasanshaya:** whose doubts
have been removed

**Chidaananda:** supreme joy

**Chirantana:** ancient, eternal

**Chitravesha:** with extraordinary dress

# D

**Daataa:** one who blesses the devotees, giver

**Daanavaari:** enemy of demons

**Daksha:** clever, expert

**Dakshaari:** enemy of 'Daksha' who was one of the ten sons of Brahmn

**Dakshinaanila:** like a (cold) breeze from South

**Dama:** taming, subdueing

**Dambha:** the thunderbolt of Indra

**Dandee:** hoding mace

**Dandodamayitaa:** punishing the defaulter

**Dapta:** proud, arrogant

**Darpahaadarpada:** who destroys pride, arrogance

**Dayaakara:** one who shows compassion, mercy

**Deerghatapaa:** one who performs penance for a very long time

**Devaadideva:** first god (originator) among the gods

**Devaangi:** god of fire

**Devaagnisukhada:** one who gives peace to gods through fire

**Devaasuramahaashraya:** one who gives great support to gods and demons

**Devasuramaheshwara:** great god of gods and demons

**Devaasureshwara:** lord of gods and demons

**Devaasuragururdeva:** great teacher of gods and demons

**Devachintaka:** one who thinks about, worries about gods

**Devdeva:** god of gods

**Devadevaatmasambhava:** one who produces god of gods

**Devadevamaya:** one who is like the god of gods

**Devagna:** one who knows gods

**Devanaatha:** master of gods

**Devapriya:** loved by gods/ favourite of gods

**Devasinha:** like a lion among gods

**Devendra:** Indra, the lord of gods

**Dhaamkara:** creator of lustre, splendour

**Dhaatreesha:** lord of the earth

**Dhaatrudhaamaa:** one who holds the universe

**Dhanaadhipa:** lord of wealth i.e. Kuber

**Dhanaagama:** giver of wealth

**Dhaneshwara:** lord of wealth

**Dhanu:** one who holds bow

**Dhanurdharo Dhanurved:** one who holds the bow and knows the science of archery

**Dhanvee:** one who holds bow

**Dhanya:** thankful

**Dharmaadhyaksha:** head of the religion

**Dharmachaaree:** one who follows Dharma i.e. religion, righteousness

**Dharmadhenu:** cow in the form of 'Dharma' i.e. virtue, right conduct

**Dharmapunja:** heap of
'Dharma'

**Dhava:** a lord

**Dheemaan:** knowledgeable

**Dhoorjati:** with a big block
of matted hair

**Dhrudha:** firm, assertive

**Dhrudhapragna:** one who has
firm knowledge

**Dhruva:** immovable

**Dhurya:** who bears the res-
ponsibility

**Dhwani:** sound, tune, note

**Dhyaanaadhaar:** one who
helps (supports) the 'yogis'
to meditate

**Dhyeya:** to be meditated,
contemplated or fit for
meditation

**Dhyumanistarani:** one who is
like sun and who protects

**Divaakara:** like the sun

**Divaspati:** like Indra, the king
of heaven

**Divyaayudha:** holder of divine
weapon

**Divya:** divine

**Doorashravaa:** one who can
hear distant sound

**Druhina:** hurting the enemies

**Drushti:** sight

**Duraadhara:** one who can be
worshipped with difficulty

**Duraasada:** difficult to obtain,
achieve

**Duratikrama:** difficult to cross

**Durga:** difficult to obtain

**Durgama:** difficult to know

**Durgneya:** difficult to know

**Durjaya:** unconquerable

**Durlabha:** difficult to achieve

**Durvaasaa:** illdressed, naked
like Durvaasaa rishi who
was a very irascible saint,
son of Atri and Ansuya
who was hard to please
and cursed many to suffer
misery and degradation. He
is also known for his anger

**Dusaha:** difficult to tolerate

**Dushkrutihaa:** destroyer of
bad deeds

**Duswapan Naashana:** destroyer of bad dreams

# E

**Ekaatmaa:** one soul

**Ekanaayaka:** one leader

**Ekbandhu:** one friend

# G

**Gaganakundaabha:** like the flower by the name of Gaganakunda

**Gahan:** deep, mysterious, incomprehensible

**Gambheera:** serious, solemn

**Ganakaaya:** principal of the group

**Ganeshwara:** leader of the group

**Gangaaplavodaka:** one who holds the flow of river ganges

**Gaureebhartaa:** husband of Gauree, Paarvati

**Gayatrivallabha:** one who likes the sacred verse of Gayatri

**Gireesha:** lord of mountains

**Girijaadhava:** husband of Paarvati

**Girirata;** one who plays on the mountain

**Gnaanagamya:** one who can be achieved through knowledge

**Gnaanamorti:** full of knowledge

**Gnaanaskando mahaaneeti:** knowledge is whose great conduct

**Gnaanavaan:** knowledgeable

**Gomaan:** rich in herds

**Gopati:** protector of earth

**Goptaa:** the protector

**Govinda:** name of Krishna, hence, like Krishna

**Greeshma:** like greeshma season, summer

**Gruhapati:** a sacrificer who maintains the sacred and perpetual fire

**Guha:** an epithet of Kaartikeya, Vishnu and Shiva

**Gunagraahaee:** one who appreciates virtues

**Gunottoma:** with best virtue

**Guru:** great, venerable, excellent, religious, teacher, might

**Guruda:** gift of the Guru

# H

**Hara:** one who destroys

**Hari:** one who destroys the sins of devotees

**Hartaa:** the destroyer

**Hansa:** the supreme soul, Brahman

**Han sagati:** stalking in a stately manner

**Havyavaaha:** like fire

**Havyavaahana:** the bearer of oblations

**Heenadosha:** faultless

**Hiranya:** shining like gold

**Hiranyagarbha:** name used for Brahmaa hence, like Brahmaa or the soul invested in a subtle body

**Hiranyakavacha:** having an armour of gold

**Hiranyaretaa:** like fire

**Hiranyavarno:** one with gold coloured skin

**Hrutpundareekamasseena:** one who has entered the heart which is like lotus

# I

**Ishas:** one who regulates, controls all

**Ishta:** dear or desired

# J

**Jagadeesha:** lord of the universe

**Jagadaadija:** one who is born first in this world

**Jagadguru:** teacher of the universe

**Jagadhvitalshee:** one who does welfare for the universe

**Jagannaatha;** lord of the universe

**Jaleshwara:** lord of the water

**Jamadagni:** like sage Jamadagni who was a descendant of Bhrigu and father of Parasuraam. He was deeply engaged in study and had obtained entire possession of Vedas

**Janaardan:** like Vishnu, Krishna

**Janaadhyaksha:** presiding over people

**Janajanmaadi:** responsible for every soul

**Janaka:** one who created the universe

**Janmaadhipa:** lord of birth

**Japya:** worth chanting

**Jaraadishanaman:** one who can remove old age

**Jatee:** one who wears matted hair

**Jatee Mundee cha Kundalee:** one who has matted hair, shaven head and wears earrings

**Jatila:** one who has matted hair

**Jatookarnya:** one who is like the sage Jatookarnya

**Jayakaalavid:** one who knows the time of victory

**Jeevitaantakaaro Nitya:** one who destroys life eternally

**Jeeviteshwara:** one who governs life

**Jitakaama:** one who has achieved victory over passions, cupid

**Jushya:** worth serving, worshipping

**Jyotirmaya:** lustrous, brilliant

# K

**Kaalaha:** destroyer of the enemy by name of 'Kaalo'

**Kaalakaaree:** one who carries out destruction

**Kaalapaksha:** one who helps destruction

**Kaalayogi:** one who gives fruits, results at a right time

**Kaamadeva:** the god of love

**Kaamapaala:** one who fulfills the wishes (of devotees)

**Kaamashaasana:** one who punishes cupid

**Kaanta:** beautiful, attractive, brilliant

**Kaaranam:** the generative cause, creator, fater

**Kaarnikaarapriya:** one who loves 'Karen' (Oleander) flowers

**Kailaasaadhipati:** lord of 'Kailas' (abode of Shiva on a peak of Himalayas)

**Kailaasa Shikharaavaasee:** residing over Kailaas mountain

**Kalaadhara:** one who holds a digit of moon

**Kalpaadi:** renovation of all things in creation

**Kalpa:** able, competent

**Kalpavruksha:** like 'Kalpa-vruksha', an imaginary tree in heaven which is supposed to satisfy all the desires of a person sitting under it

**Kalyaanagunanaamaa:** who name and qualities does welfare

**Kalyaanaprakruti:** whose nature is to do welfare

**Kamalekshana:** with beautiful eyes like lotus

**Kamandaludhara:** one holding 'Kamandala' i.e. wooden or earthern waterpot of an ascetic

**Kanakaprabhu:** as lustrous as gold

**Kanakaneekrutavaasuki:** wearing 'Vasuki' snake as a bracelet

**Kapaalee:** one who possesses skulls

**Kapilashmashru:** with tawny coloured beard and moustache

**Karanam:** the supreme being

**Karmandee:** like 'Karmandee' sage

**Kartaa:** the supreme spirit

**Kashyapa:** like sage 'Kashyapa'

**Kavi:** a wise man, thinker, omniscient

**Keertibhushana:** whose ornament is fame

**Ketu:** like 'Ketu'

**Khaga:** one who flies in the sky

**Khandaparashu:** having a battle axe which can destroy

**Khatwaangee:** one who possesses a weapon called 'Khatwaanga'

**Kireetee:** one who wears crown

**Kondandee:** one who holds bow

**Krushna:** with black neck

**Krutaagama:** creator of 'Sastras', which is a traditional doctrine, precept or scripture

**Krutaananda:** one who is happy or gives happiness or creates happiness

**Krutagna:** knowledgeable about the deeds, happenings

**Kruttivaasa:** one who wears the skin of tiger

**Kshaama:** epithet of Vishnu

**Kshamaakshetram:** origin of forgiveness

**Kshapana:** destroye.

**Kshetragna:** the supreme soul

**Kshetrapaalaka:** protector of holy places

**Kuberabandhu:** friend of 'Kuber', the god of riches

**Kumaara:** name of Kartikeya, the god of war

**Kumuda:** like a flower which gives pleasure

**Kushalaagama:** one who looks after the health and well being (of devotees)

# L

**Lalaataaksha:** having an eye on the forehead

**Lalita:** attractive, beautiful

**Lingaadhyaksha:** presiding over phalus, which is an idol of Shiva

**Lohitaatmaatanoonpaat:** like fire

**Lokabandhu:** friend of human race, people

**Lokachaaree:** one who moves about in all three worlds

**Lokagudha:** hidden in the world

**Lokakartaa:** creator of different divisions of the universe

**Lokalaavanayakartaa:** giving beauty to people

**Lokanaatha:** master of 'Loka' i.e. different divisions of the universe

**Lokapaala:** protector of universe

**Lokavarnottama:** best among all the people of all castes

**Lokaveeraagranee:** a leading hero of the world

**Lokkalpadhruk:** one who holds the world

**Lokkara:** the creator of different divisions (lokasas) of the universe

**Lokottaraskutaaloka:** whose brilliance is unbearable to people

**Lokottarasukhaalaya:** abode of best happiness

# M

**Maangalyo Mangalaavruta:**
auspicious and one who
gives benefit

**Maataamaha:** the mother of
the universe

**Maatarishwaanabhasvaana:**
like wind in the sky

**Madhurapriyadarshana:** who
looks pleasing (sweet) and
loving

**Madhyastha:** impartial,
mediator

**Maghavaan Kaushika:** muni-
ficient like Indra

**Mahaapala:** very powerful

**Mahaabhoopa:** great ruler,
sovereign

**Mahaabhuja:** with big arms

**Mahaabuddhi:** great intelligence

**Mahaadeva:** great god

**Mahaadhana:** wealthy

**Mahaadhipa:** great lord

**Mahaadhyuti:** great splendour,
brilliance

**Mahaagarbha:** who creates
great gods

**Mahaagarta:** a big throne or
veda

**Mahaahruda:** a large pool of
water

**Mahaajyotirnuttama:** best of
all and very brilliant

**Mahaakaala:** great opportune
time

**Mahaakalpa:** very able

**Mahaakopa:** very angry

**Mahaakosha:** big treasure

**Mahaakartaa:** great creator or
one who performs great
deeds

**Mahaamaaya:** with great illusion or affection

**Mahaanaada:** one who makes
big sound

**Mahaanidhi:** like a big strange

**Mahaaretaa:** very virile

**Mahaaroopa:** with great form

**Mahaashaktirmahaadhyuti:**
with great power and lustre

**Mahaatapaa:** great ascetic

**Mahaatejaa:** most brilliant,
powerful

**Mahaaveera:** great hero

**Mahaaveerya:** great heroism

**Mahaayashaa:** with great
game

**Mahaayogee:** great yogee

**Maharshikapilaachaarya:** like
sage 'Kapila'

**Maheshwara:** great god

**Maheshwaasa:** with big bow

**Maheebhartaa:** husband or
lord of earth

**Mahotsaaha:** very enthusiastic

**Mahoushadhi:** panacea,
sovereign remedy

**Manipoora:** one who fulfils
the wishes by giving pre-
cious stone

**Manobuddhi:** like mind and
intelligence

**Manojava:** as speedy as mind

**Megha:** rains i.e. one who is
like rainy season

**Mrudu:** delicate

**Mruda:** one who gives happiness

**Mrugapati:** lord of animals

**Mrugavyaadha:** hunters following Brahma who had turned himself into a deer

**Mundee:** shaven head

# N

**Naakesha:** lord of gods

**Naagabhooshana:** with ornaments of snakes

**Naagahaaradhruk:** one who wears the necklace of snakes

**Nabharava:** like rains

**Nabhogati:** who moves in the sky

**Nabhoyoni:** generating the cause for the sky, water, atmosphere

**Nadeedhara:** one who holds river

**Nagnavratadhara:** having a vow to remain naked

**Nalkaatmaa Nalkakarmakruta:** having many forms and performing many deeds

**Nakshatramaalee:** one who is wearing a garland of 'nakshatraas' i.e.27 constellations

**Naanaabhootarata:** one who lays with many beings

**Nandee:** joy and also Shiva's riding bull

**Nandeeshwara:** lord of the riding bull

**Naranaaraayanapriya:** favourite of men and god Vishnu

**Narasinh Nipaatana:** one who destroyed the pride of the one who had taken birth as 'Narasinh'

**Neelagreeva:** with black neck

**Neelakantha:** one who has black neck

**Neelalohita;** blackish blue and red (Shiva's neck is blue and 'jataa' (matted hair) are of reddish colour)

**Nidaadhastapana:** like autumn season

**Nidhi:** storage

**Niraakaara:** without disease

**Niravarananirvaara:** devoid of any sentimental bondages

**Nirahankaara:** without arrogance

**Nirantara;** perpetual, constant

**Niraatanka:** without disease

**Nirankusha:** one who does not have any control over him

**Niravadyamaayopaaya:** one who can be obtained by harmless means

**Nirleponishprapanchaatmaa:** one who remains detached from the worldly life

**Nandiskandadhara:** one who sits on the back of 'Nandi', the bull

**Naravaahana:** as epithet of Kubera, hence like Kubera

**Nata:** dancer

**Nayanaadhyaksha:** one who resides in everybody's eyes

**Nishaachara:** one who moves about at night

**Nishkalanka:** spotless

**Nishkantaka:** without enemy

**Nishreyasaan Patha:** like blessed, blissful path

**Nitya:** permanent

**Nityashaantiparaayana:** always being peaceful

**Nityasundera:** eternally beautiful

**Nirmama:** detached

**Nirmoha:** detached, without troubles

**Nirvyaarjo Vyaajaamardana:** one who is without any fraud, deceit and one who is a destroyer of frauds

**Nirvyanga:** without deformity

**Niyat Kalyaana:** constantly doing welfare

**Niyataatmaa:** one with eternal form

**Nyaayagamya:** obtained through justice

**Nyaayanirmaayakonyaayee:** judge who has created justice

**Nrutyapriyo Nityanrutya:** one who always likes to dance

# O

**Ojasvee:** possessing force of own soul or possessing valour, vitality, lustre

**Ojastejodhyutidhara:** one who is brilliant with power and valour

# P

**Panchajanya:** conch of Krishna

**Paadapassana:** one who sits near the tree

**Paanduraabha:** one with whitish lustre

**Paapahaa;** one who destroys sins

**Paarampaara:** one who emanicipates the soul from this mortal world

**Paarijaata:** name of one of the five trees of paradise

**Paavana:** sacred

**Panchayajnasamutpattis:** one from whom five 'yagnas' are produced

**Panchavinshanti tatvastha:** one who resides in twenty five elements

**Padmagarbha:** in whose lotus like heart Brahma resides

**Padmaasana:** one who resides in the hearts which are like lotuses

**Paraarthavruttivarada:** blessings for the happiness of others

**Paraashara:** like sage 'Paraashara' who was father of Vyasa and the author of a 'Smriti'

**Paramaarthaguru:** a teacher who gives 'moksha', emancipation

**Parakaaryeyka pandita;** eager to help others

**Paranjyoti:** the supreme light

**Paramaartha:** one who gives emancipation

**Paraatpara:** the supreme being

**Paramam:** excellent, greatest, supreme, prominent part

**Paramphalam:** one who gives highest fruit

**Paranjaya:** the winner of enemies

**Parantapa:** one who makes enemies suffer

**Parashwadhee:** one who holds 'Parashu', a battle axe

**Parivrudha:** the lord of all

**Parapuranjaya:** one who wins over the cities of the enemies

**Pashupati:** the lord of all the animals

**Patu:** intelligent, clever, skillful, ingenious, sagacious

**Pauraana:** sung by 'Puranas', an ancient scripture

**Pavitra:** holy, sacred

**Pinaakapaani:** the bearer of bow named 'Pinaaka'

**Pinakee:** one who holds 'Pinaka' bow

**Pingala:** the tawny coloured

**Pingalaaksha:** one with tawny colour eyes

**Poorayitaa:** one who satisfies, completes

**Poorna:** full, complete

**Pootamoorti:** sacred idol

**Praanshu:** brilliant

**Prabhanjana:** one who breaks into pieces, or stormy wind

**Prabhaakara:** brilliant, the sun

**Prabhava:** one who creates, originates everything

**Pradhaana Prabhu:** highest god

**Prakaashaatmaa Prakaashaka:** one in form of light

**Prakata:** visible

**Pramaanabhoota:** in form of measure

**Pramaanagna:** knowing the modes of proofs as a logician would

**Pramaanam:** one who judges or decides

**Pranava:** like 'Om'

**Prásannaatmaa:** delighted, satisfied soul

**Prashaantabuddhi:** one who has tranquil wisdom

**Prataptaa:** one who performs difficult penance

**Pratishthita:** celebrated, valued

**Preetimaan:** pleased

**Preetivardhana:** one who increases love

**Pretachaaree:** one who moves with ghosts

**Priyabhakta:** one who loves devotees

**Punya:** holy, meritorious

**Punyaatmaa:** pious soul

**Pulaha:** one who is like sage 'Pulaha', one of the mind-born sons of Brahmaa

**Pulastya:** one who is like sage 'Pulastya', one of the mind-born sons of Brahaa

**Punyadarshana:** seeing one who is holy, meritorious

**Punyakeerti:** one who is meritoriously famous

**Punyashravanakeertana:** it is auspicious to take the name and hear the name

**Puraatana:** ancient

**Purandara:** the destroyer of cities of enemies

**Puruhoota Purushruta:** one who performs many 'yagnas' (sacrifices) and knows 'shrutis' (sacred books)

**Purashaasana:** the destroyer of the three cities of gold, silver and iron in the sky, air and earth, built for demons by 'Maya' and these were burnt down along with demons by Shiva at the request of gods

**Purusha:** full form

**Pushkala:** best among all

**Pushkara:** a blue lotus

**Pushpalochana.** one whose eyes are like flowers

# R

**Rajanijanaka:** the creator of a dreadful night when world was destructed or pitchdark night

**Rasada:** one who knows pleasure

**Rasagna:** one who knows pleasure, delight

**Rasapriya:** one who is fond of pleasure, love, charm

**Ravilochana:** whose eyes is the sun

**Ravi:** Sun

**Ripujeevahara:** one who takes the life of enemies

**Rishi:** seer, sage, a person to whom new knowledge is revealed

**Rochishnu:** brilliant

**Ruchi:** one who has light, splendour

**Ruchiraangada:** one who wears armlets on the arms

**Rudra:** terrible, fearful

**Saadhu Saadhya:** easy for devotees to attain

**Saaksheehyakartaa:** being a witness to all he himself does not do everything

**Saamageyapriya:** one who loves to be appeased

**Saanuraaga:** having love

**Saara:** essence

**Saara Samplava:** instrumental to take out the meaning, essence of understanding

**Saaro maanadhana:** essence of all and respect is whose wealth

**Saattvika:** possessed of 'sattva' quality

**Sadaachaaree:** one who always acts truthfully

**Sadaagati:** always moving

**Sadaashiva:** always involved in doing welfare

**Sadgati:** emancipated

**Sadsanmaya:** form of truth and non-truth

**Sadyogee:** best yogiee

**Sadyoni:** cause of all

**Sagana:** together with the groups

**Sahastraarchi:** with thousand rays

**Sahastrabaahu:** with thousand hands

**Sahastrajit:** who has won victory over thousands

**Sahastramoordhaa:** with thousand heads

**Sajjaati:** creator of best races

**Sakala:** complete, full

**Sakalaadhaara:** support of all

**Sakalaagamapaaraga:** expert in vedas

**Samaadhivedya:** one who can be known through deep meditation, trance

**Samaannaaya:** similar to vedas

**Samaana:** same or one or uniform

**Samaavartta:** who revolves this world

**Samartha:** able, powerful

**Sambhaavya:** revered by all

**Samraata:** emperor

**Samvatsara:** year

**Samvatsarakara:** maker of year or time

**Sanaatana:** eternal

**Sangrahee:** one who receives kindly

**Sansaarachakrabhoota:** holding a 'chakra' which is the universe

**Saptaavara Muneeshwara:** god of seven sages and others

**Sarga:** the universe

**Sarva:** one who can take all forms

**Sarvaachaarya Manogati:** one who moves as knowledge in the minds of teachers

**Sarvaadi:** ahead of all

**Sarvaavaasa:** one who resides everywhere

**Sarvaayudhavishaarada:** one who knows use of all weapons

116

**Sarva bandha vimochana:** one who gets a person out of all the bondages

**Sarvabhoota Maheshwara:** great god of all

**Sarvadevottamottama:** very best among all gods

**Sarvadrukasinha:** like a lion who watches all

**Sarvaga:** the supreme being or one who pervades everywhere

**Sarvagochara:** looking after everyone or having everyone within bower

**Sarvakarmaalaya:** field of all actions

**Sarvalokadhruk:** one who holds all the worlds

**Sarvalokaprajaapati:** lord of all the people and 'lokaas' worlds

**Sarvapaapharohara:** one who destroys everyone's sins

**Sarvapramaana Samvaadee:** in harmony with all kinds of measures

**Sarvarturaparivartaka:** one who changes all seasons

**Sarvasaadhana:** one who achieves everything

**Sarvasattva:** support of all

**Sarvasattvaavalambana:** support of all animate and inanimate objects

**Sarvashaasana:** one who governs everybody

**Sarvashaastra Bhrutanvara:** best among those who know all 'shastras'

**Sarvashaastraprabhanjana:** destroyer of all shastras

**Sarvaroopa:** with all forms

**Sarvashuddhi:** one who purifies all

**Sarvataapanas:** like the sun who gives heat to all

**Sarvayoni:** originator of all

**Sarvesha:** god of all

**Sarveshwara:** god of everybody

**Satkruti:** one who performs good deed

**Satpathaachara:** having truthful conduct

**Sattvavaachana:** carrier of 'sattva'

**Sattvavaana:** storage of virtues

**Satya:** truth

**Satyakeerti:** with genuine fame

**Satyaparaakrama:** with truthful action

**Satya Satyapara:** in the nature of truth and always anxious for truth

**Satyavratsmahaatyaagee:** one who observes vow of truth and is a great sacrificer

**Savitaa:** sun

**Setu:** the sacred syllable 'Om'

**Shaakalya:** like 'Shaakalya' sage, an ancient grammarian who is supposed to have arranged the 'pada' text of the 'Rigveda'

**Shaakhya:** like 'Kartikeya'

**Shaanta:** quiet, peaceful

**Shaantabhadra:** doing welfare for peaceful people

**Shaastaa:** ruler

**Shaastaa Valvasvato Yama:** ruling through yama, son of sun

**Shaila:** like a mountain

**Shakra:** Indra

**Shambara:** in form of water

**Shakrapramaathee:** one who has defeated Indra

**Shalabha:** one who roams everywhere

**Shambhu:** one who looks after the welfare of devotees

**Shani:** like 'Shani'

**Sharabha:** one who has taken 'Avataara' of Sharabha i.e. young elephant or a fabulous animal said to have 8 legs and stronger than a lion or camel or a locust

**Sharanam:** one who gives protection to all

**Sharanya:** worth resorting to

**Shareeraashritavatsala:** one who loves animate and inanimate objects who are dependent on him

**Sharva:** one who brings an end to everything

**Sharvareepati:** like moon

**Shatrujitchhatrutaapana:** one who wins the enemies and makes them suffer

**Sheeghraga:** one who goes speedily

**Sheeghranaashana:** one who destroys speedily

**Shikhandee Kavachee Shoolee:** one who has matted hair, armour and trident

**Shikhisaarathi:** one whose charioteer is fire

**Shikhishreeparvatapriya:** having affection for 'Shree Parvata' of Kartikeya

**Shipvishta:** pervaded by rays

**Shishiraatmaka:** like 'Shishira' season

**Shishkeshta:** worshipped by scholars

**Shishu:** child

**Shiva:** one who looks after welfare

**Shivaalaya:** a place of welfare

**Shivagnaanarata:** absorbed in self knowledge

**Siddha:** one who has achieved

**Siddha Vrundaara Vandita:** one who is revered by gods and Siddhas

**Siddhi:** one who has achieved

**Siddhida:** one who gives accomplishment, fulfillment

**Siddhisaadhana:** one who is instrumental for accomplishment

**Shobhana:** decorative, beautiful

**Shokanaashana:** destroyer of sorrow

**Shreekantha:** with beautiful voice

**Shreemaan:** one with wealth

**Shreya:** best, desirable

**Shrutimaan:** one who knows vedas

**Shrutiprakaasha:** brilliant because of knowledge of vedas

**Shubhaanga:** beautiful body

**Shubhada:** one who gives goodness

**Shubhakartaa:** one who does good, welfare

**Shubhanaamaashubhaswayam:** one whose name is auspicious and who himself is felicitous.

**Shuchi:** pious

**Shuchismita:** with pure, holy smile

**Shuddhaatmaa:** pure soul

**Soorya:** sun

**Shuddhavigraha:** who spreads purity

**Skanda:** name of Kartikeya, son of Shiva

**Skandaguru:** teacher of Kartikeya Swami

**Smashaananilaya:** one who resides in crematorium

**Snigdha Prakruiti Dakshina:** with loving and clever nature

**Snehakrutaagama:** who lovingly creates 'shastras'

**Soma:** nectar or a ray of light or like a moon

**Somapa:** who drinks 'soma rasa' (juice)

**Somarata:** having affection for moon

**Sookshma:** minute, subtle

**Sooryataapana:** who makes sun shine

**Sootrakaara:** author of aphorisms

**Soumya:** gentle, mild

**Spashtaakshara:** as clear words as 'Om'

**Srashtaa;** creator

**Stavapriya:** who is fond of praise

**Stavya:** praiseworthy

**Sthaanada:** one who gives position

**Sthapati Sthira:** permanent architect

**Sthavira:** old man

**Sthavistha:** greatest, very strong

**Stragvee:** one who wears garland

**Stuta:** one who is praised

**Stutya:** praiseworthy

**Subhaga:** wealthy, prosperous

**Subrahmanya:** well versed in sacred knowledge

**Sudhaapati:** lord of nectar

**Sudhee:** having best knowledge

**Sugata:** well bestowed or an epithet of Buddha

**Sukara:** with beautiful hands

**Sukhaanila:** like comforting breeze

**Sukhi:** giver of happiness

**Sukeerti:** good fame

**Sukumaara:** very tender

**Sulabha:** easily available

**Sulochana:** with beautiful eyes

**Sumatirvidhvaana:** with best intellect and knowledge

**Sumukha:** with beautiful face

**Suneeti:** embodiment of good conduct

**Sunishpanna:** one who can produce well

**Suparna:** well winged or having beautiful leaves

**Suprateeka:** with beautiful face

**Supreeta:** one who is beloved

**Suraadhyaksha:** principal deity among gods

**Surabhi:** like spring season

**Suragana:** assembly of gods

**Surasattama:** best among gods

**Suresha:** god of gods

**Susharana:** a good place for refuge

**Sushenassurashatruhaa:** one who defeats the enemies of gods with the help of a large battalion of soldiers

**Sutantu:** one who spreads or covers well

**Swabhaava Bhadra:** having a nature to do good

**Suvratashhoora:** like sun and fulfilling the vow of protecting devotees

**Suveera:** best hero

**Swaadhishthaanapadaashraya:** one who emancipates yogees

**Swadharmaa:** one who follows his own religion

**Swadhruta:** self supportive

**Swaksha:** with beautiful eyes

**Swarbandhu:** colleagues from heaven

**Swargata:** residing in heaven

**Swargasvara:** one tha can be heard in the heaven

**Swaramaya svana:** one who produces all the seven notes of music

**Swastida:** doing welfare for devotees

**Swastikrut:** doing welfare for all

**Swayamjyotistanujyoti:** self illuminated with subtle light

# T

**Taraka:** one who carries the devotees through

**Taarkshya:** an epithet of eagle, one who is form of eagle

**Tamistrahaa:** one who removes the darkness

**Tamohara:** one who removes the darkness

**Tarasvee:** speedy

**Tantuyardhana:** one who extends, expands the world

**Tapa:** Penance

**Tapaswee:** one who is practising penance

**Tattvam:** the real nature of the human soul or the material world as being identical with the supreme spirit pervading the universe

**Tattvavit:** one who knows supreme spirit

**Tigmaanshu:** with sharp rays

**Teerthankara:** the writer of 'Sgastras'

**Tejoraashirmahaamani:** like a big jewel which shines as accumulated store of light

**Trayeetanu:** one whose body is like three vedas

**Tridashaadhipa:** presiding over thirty three gods

**Trilochana:** with three ways

**Trilokapa:** the protector of three worlds

**Trilokesha:** lord of three worlds

**Trishoolee:** one who holds trident

**Trivargassargasaddhana:** one who has created the world in form of religion, wealth and desires

**Teerthadeva Shivaalaya:** like benevolent gods of holy places

**Teerthanaamaa:** one who is as holy as 'Teertha'

**Tejomaya:** luminous

**Tejomaya Dhyutidhara:** brilliant and beautiful

**Trividya:** one who has three types of knowledge

**Tryakshal:** with three eyes

**Trambakal:** with three eyes

**Tumbhaveena:** one who has 'Veena' made out of gourd, pumpkin

**Turhta:** satisfied

# U

**Udaara Keerti:** with big fame

**Udyogee:** diligent, active

**Ugra:** hot tempered, angry

**Unnadhra:** one who fastens sinfuls

**Unmattavesha Prachhana:** secretly clad as a mad man

**Ushna:** hot, warm

**Upaplava:** a portent or natural phenomenon foreboding evil

**Uttara:** one who carries through, delivers

# V

**Vachaspati:** lord of all the knowledge

**Vaagesha:** lord of speech

**Vaalakhilya:** like sage named 'Vaalakhilya'

**Vaamadeva:** beautiful looking god

**Vaaraaha Shrungadhruka- shrungee:** one who has the horns of boar

**Vaayuvaahana:** one who drives wind

**Vairanchya:** like the son of Brahmaa

**Vaiyaghradhurya:** one who wears the skin of tiger

**Vajrahasta:** having lightning in hand like Indra

**Varaanga:** with beautiful body

**Varada:** one who gives blessings

**Varaguna:** with best virtue

**Varasheela:** one who has best character

**Varesha:** best god

**Varnaashramaguru:** teacher of castes and 'ashramas'

**Vasanto Madhava:** like the splendour of spring season

**Vasishtha:** like the celebrated saga 'Vasishtha'

**Vasu:** wealthy, good

**Vasudhaamaa:** place of wealth

**Vasuprada:** one who gives wealth

**Vasuretaa:** one with golden fire

**Vasushravaa:** like hearing sweet things

**Vatsala:** dear

**Vaya:** a weaver

**Vedaanga:** part of veda

**Vedaanta Sandoha:** one who knows the meaning, gist of Vedaantaas

**Vedakara:** creator of Vedas

**Vedha Vidhaataa:** creator of universe, organiser of uni- verse and supporter of universe

**Vedashaastraarthatatvagna:** one who knows the deep meaning of veda and shaastraas

**Veda Vinmuni:** sage who knows vedas

**Vedya:** worth knowing

**Veera:** powerful

**Veeraasana Vidhi:** one who brings conduct on battle- field

**Veerabhadra:** name of a powerful hero created by Shiva from his matted hair

**Veerachoodaamani:** shining among the heroes like the jewel worn on the head

**Veereshwara:** lord of heroes

**Veeryavaan Veeryakovida:** heroic and clever at bravery

**Veetabhaya:** without fear

**Veetaraaga:** ascetic

**Vegeeplaranas:** going every- where with speed

**Vetta:** one who knows

**Vibhu:** pervasive

**Vibudhaagravarshrestha:** bet- ter than the foremost gods

**Vichkshana:** one who has special knowledge

**Vidheyaatmaa:** one who has control over soul, aatmaa

**Vidhvattama:** great scholar

**Vidrumacchavi:** shining like coral

**Vidyaaraashi:** accumulation of all 'vidyas', knowledge

**Vidyosha:** lord of knowledge

**Vigaala:** one who would emancipate

**Vigatajwara:** one who removes all fevers, pains, afflictions, grief

**Vigneya:** one who has special knowledge

**Vijaya:** victory

**Vijitaatmaa:** one who has won the soul

**Vikartaa:** one whose designs are wonderful, variegated, strange

**Vikramonnata:** mightest of all

**Vikruta:** one who performs special acts

**Vimala:** pure

**Vimalodaya:** one who does welfare or one who purifies

**Vimochana:** one who releases devotees from their sins

**Vineetaatmaa:** well educated soul

**Viraama:** place for all to rest

**Viranchee:** brahman or like Brahmaa

**Virakta:** free from worldly attachments

**Virochana:** brilliant, lustrous

**Viroopa:** one with special form

**Virropaaksha:** with ill looking, ugly eyes

**Vishaalaaksha:** with big eyes

**Vishaakha:** like Kartikeya

**Vishaarada:** a scholar

**Vishamaaksha:** one with uneven eyes

**Vishanpati:** lord of the universe

**Vishishta:** best

**Vishnu prajaapaala:** like Vishnu who is a protector of people

**Vishnukandharapaatana:** one who could bend the neck of Vishnu

**Vishoka:** without sorrow, grief

**Vishtarashravaa:** like Vishnu

**Vishwaavaasa:** residing in entire universe

**Vishwabhartaa:** supporter of universe

**Vishwabhojana:** eating away the world at the time of 'pralaya'

**Vishwadeepti:** light of the universe

**Vishwagaalava:** like Gaalava sage in the world who was the pupil of Viswaamitra

**Vishwagarbha:** in whom entire universe resides

**Vishwagoptaa:** supporting the universe

**Vishwakarmaa:** expert in the creation of universe

**Vishwakartaa:** creator of the universe

**Vishwaamitra:** a friend of all

**Vishwam:** universe

**Vishwambhareshwara:** one who protects, supports the universe

**Vishwamoorti:** embodiment of the universe

**Vishwasaha:** creator of the universe

**Vishwata Sanvruta:** prevailing everywhere

**Vishwavaahana:** one who runs the world

**Vishwavibhushana:** like an ornament of the universe

**Vishwesha:** lord of the universe

**Vishwotpatti:** creator of the universe

**Viyogaatmaa:** one who can be known by special yoga

**Vrushaanka;** with the sign of bull

**Vrushado Vrushavardhana:** one who gives virtues and propagates virtues

**Vyaaghra Charmaambara:** one who wears tiger's skin

**Vrusha Vaahana:** one who sits on bull or one who has bull as transport

**Vyaaghralochana:** having eyes like a tiger

**Vyaalaakalpa:** one who has ornaments of snakes

**Vyaalee:** one who holds snakes

**Vyaapti:** one who resides everywhere

**Vyaasmoorti:** like sage Vyaasa

**Vyanganaashana:** destroyer of deformity

**Vyavasaaya:** perseverance, determination, action

**Vyavasthaana:** arrangement, settlement, decision

**Vyadhoraska:** with broad chest

# Y

**Yagna:** an act of worship, devotional act

**Yashodhana:** one who is rich with fame

**Yogaathyakshas:** one who presides over 'yoga'

**Yogapaara:** expert in yoga

**Yogavidyogee:** yogee who is expert in yoga

**Yogiyogya:** proper or qualified for yoga

**Yugaadikrudyugaavarta:** one who started an era and runs it

**Yugaavaha:** one who directs the age of the world

**Yuktirunnatakoti:** one with great fame